CW00519668

Journey From Venice

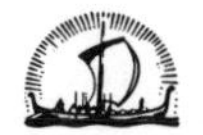

RUTH
CRACKNELL

Journey
From Venice

A MEMOIR

VIKING

Viking
Penguin Books Australia Ltd
487 Maroondah Highway, PO Box 257
Ringwood, Victoria 3134, Australia
Penguin Books Ltd
Harmondsworth, Middlesex, England
Penguin Putnam Inc.
375 Hudson Street, New York, New York 10014, USA
Penguin Books Canada Limited
10 Alcorn Avenue, Toronto, Ontario, Canada M4V 3B2
Penguin Books (NZ) Ltd
Cnr Rosedale and Airborne Roads, Albany, Auckland, New Zealand
Penguin Books (South Africa) (Pty) Ltd
5 Watkins Street, Denver Ext. 4, 2094, South Africa
Penguin Books India (P) Ltd
11, Community Centre, Panchsheel Park, New Delhi 110 017, India

First published by Penguin Books Australia Ltd, 2000

1 3 5 7 9 10 8 6 4 2

Design and digital imaging by Ellie Exarchos, Penguin Design Studio
Cover photography by Tracey Schramm, Garry Moore, Michel Brouet and The Photo Library
Typeset in 13/18.5 Centaur by Midland Typesetters, Maryborough, Victoria
Printed and bound in Australia by Australian Print Group, Maryborough, Victoria

National Library of Australia
Cataloguing-in-Publication data:

Cracknell, Ruth.
Journey from Venice.

ISBN 0 670 88614 9.

1. Phillips, Eric. 2. Loss (Psychology). 3. Husbands – Death – Psychological aspects. 4. Grief. 5. Bereavement – Psychological aspects. I. Title.

155.937

www.penguin.com.au

To Anna, Jane and Jonathan

Contents

ACKNOWLEDGEMENTS

I am indebted to friends and colleagues who were of assistance and support to me during the period this book was forming in my mind and, subsequently, during the course of writing it. I hope they will forgive me for merely listing them considering how vital this assistance was. In no particular order then, Maev O'Meara, Phillip Moore, Dr Margot Harris, Philomena Moore, John Rogers, Susan Rogers, Kirrily Nolan, Lisa McKimmie, Julieanne Newbould, Ron Blair, Jennifer Hagan, and Petrea King of the Quest for Life Foundation.

My children, Anna Phillips, Jane Moore and Jonathan Phillips, assisted with details that I had overlooked, and have earned my deepest gratitude for this invasion of their privacy. It has been willingly accepted, and I trust will prove no burden. They and I were comforted and encouraged at all times during Eric's illness by the nursing staff and medical specialists at the Sydney Adventist Hospital and by the director and all staff at the Mount Wilga Private Hospital and Rehabilitation Centre.

In Venice we were deeply grateful for the care and attention of the medical staff at Ospidale Civile San Giovanni e Paolo, in particular the Primario of Internal Medicine, Dr Gabriele Bittolo Bon. Our thanks, also, to the Australian Consul in Rome, Charles Farrugia, and his dedicated staff, who were a positive force during difficult times.

Finally, thanks, and again thanks, to my literary agent, Barbara Mobbs, and my editor Bryony Cosgrove – not least for the laughs along the way.

memento mori

A Funeral

The house wakes. She lies there listening for awhile – reluctant to take the first step. Merely getting out of bed today seems beyond her. The past three months have depleted her.

But it is not just that. The day itself has no predecessor, is shrouded … an isolated fragment …

Shrouded or not no amount of lying in bed will make it go away.

On the morning of the opening night of a play I have always risen with a sense of something ominous surrounding me. More than nerves. More important than nerves, somehow. When I make the bed on that day there is a little ritual, the same words running round my mind – 'When I fall into you tonight it will be over.'

The foolishness sustains me somehow.

Absurd to be thinking these words today. They belittle the occasion.

I remain in bed as long as I can, postponing any ritual. Where is the cat? Taken herself to the basket she rejected two years ago probably, and which she has scarcely left since Monday night.

It is Friday.

The clear, treble twittering in the second bedroom announces Celeste's entry into the day. Celeste, the youngest grandchild, and Madeleine, the eldest, along with their mother, my first born, have been staying with me.

I hear them wandering into the bathroom, the kitchen.

Then Anna is at my bedroom door. 'Do you want tea, Mum?'

'No. No. I'm getting up.'

Which I do, in a moment. Hug the children, on the way to the kitchen ...

The tea and the cereal and the toast and the

clearing up and the showers and the dressing (special outfits waiting) – it all proceeds, moves them forward. Someone arrives to take Celeste away for the day; my son, Jonathan, arrives with his partner, Lisa; my other daughter, Jane, and her husband, Phillip, with their two girls; and Anna's husband, John, with their two boys.

Five children here now. Sons-in-law; Lisa; my two daughters; my son. The men suited. Formal.

Grandchildren pick bunches of wattle from the tree he and I planted a couple of years ago and which drove him to distraction with its Jack in the Beanstalk propensities. But such a bloomer of a tree! It is in full flood this July high day of sunshine and wind.

I worry that one of the boys is not warmly enough dressed. 'He needs a jumper, for heaven's sake!'

The doorbell rings again and again. Flowers are still arriving.

Through it all the women proceed to apply make-up. Madeleine's hair is being arranged. Three generations stand at the bathroom mirror.

Forty-one years on.

Four reflections.

Four similars.

Then all but my three children are gone. We will travel together. The four who journeyed to Venice – and back.

Incongruously, I am sitting at the dining-room table in front of a typewriter trying to read my daughter's handwriting – 'This is ridiculous. Why am I doing this now?' – as the knock at the door announces Kristian's arrival.

'Our car's here. Don't worry. He's early.'

I finish typing the words Anna will be reading later.

One more glance in the bathroom mirror and we gather at the door. I look at my children and not for the first time marvel at their fortitude. I am bereft and overwhelmingly proud at the same time.

Minutes later they are driving along the M2, Jonathan

next to Kristian, she with her daughters either side. Silence till –

'I feel sick!'

Why had they all forgotten Anna's fatal propensity for car sickness.

'Don't vomit on me!'

Kristian nervously states the obvious. 'I know we can't stop here!'

'Why didn't you sit in the front seat?' from Jonathan – equally in the line of fire.

'I'll be all right!'

Jane, quite safe, gazes out her window.

This day is impossible to anchor in any identifiable reality. No template.

She seems to be outside herself. If she looks through the window she has the impression of her actual self accompanying them. An Arthur Boyd bride.

Veil flying.

The motorway safely, if nervously, negotiated, they are approaching the Bridge. It is one of Sydney's stunning days – sunny, harbour scintillating, stiff breeze cutting through, making flags perform prettily.

She realises they are very early –

'Kristian, pull up near Government House.'

The car stops. Anna gratefully escapes, Jonathan next. He is carrying a Bible. An unfamiliar sight. He is to read 1 Corinthians 13 – 'Though I speak with the tongues of men and of angels, and have not love, I am become as sounding brass, or a tinkling cymbal.' He paces up and down towards the Conservatorium, reading, mouthing. Walking in the opposite direction, towards Government House, Anna is rehearsing her words. Unable to contribute anything this day, Jane stands close, with her, near the car. Kristian is standing diagonally opposite, on the other side of the car, gazing at Macquarie Street. They are the figures added to an architectural drawing to give it a sense of purpose and proportion. Or is it a crane shot in a movie? Precisely geometric when the pacers stop. Draw the lines.

Everyone feeling sick as they get back in the car. A slow drive edges them along Phillip Street and finally into King Street, where they pull up outside St James'. People are still streaming in ...

I see Ann. June. Jenny, wearing green gloves – like St Patrick's Day. Kirrily with all the staff – twenty of them – clustered around her. She will be reading one of the Sonnets. Garry stands apart, reading a handful of notes. He is to present the eulogy, written by Geoffrey.

It is approaching noon. I begin to feel anxious, my theatrical punctuality to the fore. Then, suddenly, there are the grandchildren in the porch, as the last of the stragglers move inside. Someone marshals the children, and they and the wattle disappear as noon chimes.

The rector, Richard Hurford, appears, splendid in full vestments, and we finally leave the car and mount the steps. We are greeted, form up behind him – I am with Jane, arms linked, hands crushing, the other two behind, as the music surrounds us and we proceed.

Too slowly for my taste. 'Faster clip, Richard!' (I cannot stop directing proceedings.) We enter a packed church. Full house. I am delighted – and somehow surprised. Why? Because I've always been the star? We are surrounded by people – a crush of people; there are waves and waves of sound. I am drowning ...

Mysteriously, silkily, the organ slides from its soaring Processional into a simple twenties ballad.

'What was that! Did you hear that?'

If you were the only girl in the world
And I were the only boy ...

It lingers for a few bars, then it is gone – just a wisp.

And the service begins.

I kneel, rise, slip in and out of reality, as this most beautiful of services moves through its stages. I know how good it is, fuss if it seems to drag for a moment; am at times caught up in an unbearable emotion; but mostly it is all happening to someone else.

Where is Ruth? Where has she gone? Who will find her? Who will soothe her now?

I have one clear recollection – the choir gently singing the John Rutter – 'The Lord bless you and keep you; the Lord make his face to shine upon you and be gracious unto you; the Lord lift up the light of his countenance upon you and give you peace' – while I stare at a coffin heaped with iris and the wattle.

And then it is over. The last hymn thunders

forth as the coffin is carried high, high, between the silent pews.

He is followed by his wife, his children, his grandchildren – his tribe. Out, out ... through the door ... out into the porch ...

... and the bells are peeling and the wind is screaming and it is pelting with rain and Bill Orr is pouring confetti over me and I am bursting with joy as I hang onto my husband. Ruth and Eric. Bride and groom. Photographers snapping, everyone laughing, a huge umbrella held over us, the wind snatching words away. It is icy, but we do not care. Three weeks to get ready for a wedding and we two are flying high. We're delicious! We're the tops!

What we do not know – how can we? (we would not believe it anyway) – what we do not know, he and I, is that nearly forty-one years stretch before us.

'Eric! Forty-one years! Can you believe that! Forty-one years! What bliss!'

Or that the forty-one years will be ending right here on another July day.

When the weather will be fairer.

The day bleaker.

Forty-one years.

With the speed of light . . .

Part One

Your time is not come;
love and death have their fatalities, and strike
home one time or other.
You'll pay for all one day ...

The Beaux' Stratagem
George Farquhar

At last we are in the taxi – speeding along the M2. All I am conscious of is the two of us holding hands and breathing very deeply. Will we ever get out of this manic cycle of too much work and too many deadlines? Resolve: talk about this in Venice.

Eric's six-day working week was showing no signs of easing. And my last few years had been punishing, with unforeseen developments and season extensions throwing what had seemed a reasonable schedule into near chaos. Certainly, I had no idea of the demands of a book tour. With *A Biased Memoir,* I flew all over the country. *A Little Night Music* had a return season in Melbourne, and *Vita and Virginia* went on tour.

Altogether too much for an ageing diseuse. There were one or two indications that I was pushing it ... When the main tour of *Vita and Virginia* was over, Jennifer Hagan and I flew into Sydney. Eric was to meet us. As I walked towards baggage collection I began to feel very ill. Ill in an unfamiliar way. I called out to Jenny, who was ahead, and I remember being helped towards a thoroughly alarmed Eric. There was much to-ing and fro-ing, our small travelling company endeavouring to render assistance as discreetly as possible in the circumstances – a difficult operation when a task as simple as obtaining a glass of water at Sydney Airport proved impossible for even this talented crew. If one's life depended upon it there would, I fear, be many sad endings. As I wafted in and out of my interesting state, Eric was white with anxiety. The upshot proved not too terrible. A sudden, and completely untypical, surge of blood pressure, finally sorted out with medication.

There was another incident in Perth towards the end of the book tour. Eric had flown over as soon as I was free of speeches and signings. We had time with friends; civilised lunches, arranged for us, as usual, whenever we are in Perth. I remember, at one of these, Sister Veronica Brady stating firmly that she was completely undersexed. A pebble tossed into a pond. The table paused for a moment to ponder this – digest the information – before returning with vigour to its *School For Scandal* musings and revelations. I was delighted by her exquisite timing, thought what a useful state this was in a nun. I could feel myself beginning to envy a life of such singular focus ...

And in an instant I am floating away from the table, silk veil billowing; pacing the cloisters to the accompaniment of plainsong; free of decisions; early to bed, very early to rise; certain of right and wrong; responsive only to silver bell – quiet, at peace ...

Back at the table, Sister Veronica's no-nonsense appearance, shrewd intelligence, absence of any indication of her calling, beyond, perhaps, a tiny cross at her throat, punctured my medieval daydream and returned me sharply to my imperfect human state.

After Perth, we were to spend a few days at Heytesbury Stud, at the invitation of Janet Holmes à Court, where we could relax in complete comfort before heading south to Margaret River – our final destination. Seduced by our surroundings, we decided to stay for the week – eating, reading, sleeping, walking, sipping, staring into space. It seemed perfect, and was, until I woke in the middle of the night with the room spinning. Next day's trip to a medical centre diagnosed a middle-ear infection. More medication and complete quiet ordered until things settled. By now, Eric was stealing sidelong glances, waiting for the next development. I was aware how focused he was on me, anxiety niggling …

Why was I not watching him?

It is Christmas, 1997. We are all present on the back verandah. He sits at one end of the table, I at the other, and it is the usual chaos and tumbling and rolling and coming and going of platters and talk and noise and sudden silences. Family Christmases everywhere – if you are lucky, as we are. Fortune rides high this year.

Only later, Anna remarks, 'Dad looks as though he's disappearing ...'

I am not noticing anything. Too busy drawing breath before the onslaught of the next three months. He, too, will be flat out – looking at a re-organization of our business. A tricky manoeuvre of pulling back to the Crows Nest framing shop where it all started. Manageable. Less stress on him. We are aiming for a more relaxed lifestyle, more time together, more breaks. Our reward. Not that either of us has the slightest desire for complete retirement. We are united in this. Just pulling back a little. Luxury.

Our taxi deposits us at International Departures. We are in the hell of the airport. People, people, people. It is bewildering, exhausting, but also, as ever, very exciting.

It seems an eternity, but at last we are in the Qantas lounge. Baggage has been sent all the way to Venice, money has been changed, we are sitting down, and at last we have time to look at one another. We are smiling! We are two conspirators! We have done it! Actually done it! Not a phone in sight. No one to talk to but ourselves, and we can be silent all the way to Venice if we want. No more problems; everything taken care of.

We carry impressive itineraries from our travel agent, assuring us of a smooth journey all the way. No stopover has been sought or advised, and someone, we read, will meet us at Rome and escort us to Alitalia, where we will board their flight for the short hop to Venice. Very smooth, very simple. We are to relax.

On QF1, I am reading Donna Leone's *Death at La Fenice,* the perfect introduction to Venice. No one else captures so succinctly the everyday life of the Serene City; no one else captures that particular devotion of the Venetians to their city, nor the faint contempt felt by them towards any not similarly blessed.

Eric begins the latest Linda La Plante.

Plane trips are plane trips are plane trips ... Bangkok is reached. We are to change planes. We wander aimlessly for a time. We board the new plane, the heat clutching at us. We take our seats. I start yet another sketchy diary.

MARCH 27: An ominous wait on the ground stretching to two hours. It is more than likely we shall miss the connection to Venice. We endeavour to dismiss from our minds the difficulties that little delay may bring with it.

MARCH 28: Rome airport. No escort in sight. Confusion everywhere. Is getting through the barriers here worse than elsewhere? Assuredly. A milling throng trying to escape through two tiny openings manned by officials who seem in no hurry at all to begin the day's work – let alone get through it. Their pace, when they begin, is leisurely. Europeans swan through the third opening.

Utter chaos. No one advancing. We begin to move at a snail's pace and finally, finally, we are through. No hope of making the connecting flight, so we start the agonizing business of trying to let Venice know we are delayed two hours. Eric, as usual, in these circumstances, leading the way, calming me down, using his brain. Finally, an airport official makes the call for us, reading the details from my scrap of paper. (We are to discover later that no message got through. Perhaps he would have performed any charade to rid himself of the crazed woman who stopped just short of flinging herself at his feet and licking his shoes.)

Draw a veil here over the absence of any welcome at Venice, the taxi trip along the canals, myself in a temper, our female courier outrageous. The delay, it seems, has presented *her* with a problem as she will be running late for her next arrival if she fulfils her obligations to us by escorting us to our door. It is her intention to dump us at a wharf – any wharf – and then make your own way, sweethearts! Eric is trying to take the odd photograph. I am snarling. My suggestion of chucking money at her works – up to a point. She graciously decides to lead the way to our apartment. 'Leading the way' for this courier consists of galloping ahead through the maze that is Venice, with me doing my best to keep her in sight as I struggle behind with the cabin bags. Eric is bringing up the rear, wheeling two cases. Up and over bridge after bridge. Our 'guide' disappears swiftly. We are in *Alice in Wonderland,* with a particularly nasty white rabbit leading us a merry dance, flicking round corners, and only occasionally bothering to check if anyone is panting behind her in the maze. I keep having to retrace steps to see if Eric is still with us. I am at last deposited, metaphorically, into the arms of the agent for the flat where we will be staying for the next three weeks. Our tormentor vanishes into thin air. I send the agent to help a completely exhausted Eric. Eventually they return. We have arrived at San Marco 998, Corte Gregolini.

The agent for the flat is Nicole Payet. I look at her properly for the first time.

There is no flicker of recognition here from either of us. Where is the snapshot of this moment? I would peruse it again and again. Where the light? Why no sword? The moment is completely undistinguished, unmarked ... it should be mandatory for guardian angels to carry identification.

Nicole is from the Seychelles, but has lived in Venice for many years and is married to a Venetian who is in love with the Seychelles. He cannot wait to retire there, so all their earnings are headed in that direction. I hope they are strolling along sandy beaches right now …

Super efficient, Nicole shows us round this small but eminently satisfactory living space. We complete our business and she departs, leaving us with all contact numbers, including her mobile.

We discover we are in a basement flat, which no Venetian, of course, would contemplate laying head to rest in, but it suffices for our time here – always provided there is no sudden aqua alta. We are innocent of such things, anyway. Our flat is on the corner of a crumbling sixteenth-century building, and there are four canals intersecting beneath the windows. Gondolas are sliding past as we begin to unpack, the gondoliers making their strange call as they round corners. Sometimes they sing – the most delightful sound in the world, we think. It is topped suddenly by the crashing, awesome noise of bells! We cannot believe this glorious pealing. It is right on top of us. We need to share it, so in the middle of unpacking, we pick up the phone – find Jane at home. We hold the phone out the window, and Jane in Sydney hears Venice's bells as clearly as if they were resounding from the next street. She is suitably amazed. She is hearing the bells that will be ringing the changes through our time here ...

It is impossible to concentrate on unpacking.

Look out one window, there is a bridge that backs onto a hotel beloved of the tourist industry. We will see many come and go from this hotel. First, their luggage will be piled up in a water taxi. Someone – from Texas? – will stand on the bridge, and under his wife's instructions photograph the pile of luggage beneath, in the centre of which may rest her vanity case; then the taxis will arrive to take the human cargo, their two days in Venice faithfully recorded, their heads stuffed with bewildering information and images that may fade just a little as their plane lands at the next airport.

Out of the side windows we can just glimpse another bridge spanning the nearer offshoot canal. This is where the major traffic jams occur, but how pleasantly, how delightfully, accompanied as they are by musical voices, and the absence of abuse and car horns.

We do not finish the unpacking – we simply close the door of our apartment behind us, and with not a little sense of adventure go through the impressive front door and out into our tiny corte. As with dozens of other cortes in Venice, it is small and enclosed by tall buildings, most of them dating from the sixteenth or seventeenth century. There is a well in the centre, and when we look above the enclosed gardens and jumble of buildings beyond the corte, we can see the splendid angel atop the Campanile, revolving almost imperceptibly. Every time we emerge from the front door he will present a different aspect. He is the first thing we look at. Our corte is distinguished by having one corner taken up by a police station, which adds, we feel, a certain sense of security to our dwelling. I am not sure why we should feel this – we seldom see the police, they are invariably plain clothed, carry files and briefcases and firmly shut their street door behind them before mounting to the first floor. A pile of small rocks would be required to gain their attention.

We take the narrow passageway out of Corte Gregolini and turn right – our aim that first afternoon to familiarize ourselves with the route to San Marco. Our first glimpse is heart stopping, even in a Piazza crowded with tourists. It is fair time at San Marco – popcorn vendors for the pigeons, music from the small orchestra, which is probably, even on that first day, playing Strauss; there is selling and horse trading on all sides, and children and adults are turning themselves into pantomime characters with very silly hats. School groups, tour groups – every conceivable nationality – cameras pointed up, down, sideways. I always pity the photographer, eye resolutely clamped to view finder, hardly a moment to sit and stare. This is the reason for our extended stay. There *will* be time for staring.

We get our bearings in the Piazza, map out an easy plan for Sunday, and walk to the Grand Canal, loving the cheek-by-jowl bobbing of gondolas and the view straight across to Giudecca and San Giorgio Maggiore. We do not share Ruskin's view of San Giorgio – 'It is impossible to conceive a design more gross, more barbarous, more childish in conception, more servile in plagiarism, more insipid in result, more contemptible under every point of rational regard.' Perhaps this luminous Saturday the weather is better.

We dine that evening at a restaurant we aim not to return to.

Our flat contains enough utensils for the preparation of meals when economic realities occasionally intrude. There is a toaster I would willingly steal if only it were possible to rid oneself of a lifetime's moral quibblings in these matters. This is an ancient toaster with a timer that is switched on for five or six minutes. Two slices of bread reside in a basket device, and the bread is gradually dried to present toast so perfect that every morning is a marvel. The basket is then carried to the table, and I have been looking for something engineered in similar fashion ever since. Not to be found. It is far too primitive.

The bathroom presents the only worry, as plumbing seems dubious in the extreme, an ever-present possibility of canal rising up through plug-hole or lavatory bowl.

There is ample storage for luggage, and enough, if temperamental, heating.

I will come to love the ritual of closing the

shutters at night and opening them early in the morning, never too sure what eye-to-eye contact may happen as gondola or barge is manoeuvred skilfully past.

MARCH 29: Early morning in the Piazza. The only time. Free of the hordes. Beautiful spring weather. Opportunity to stand quietly and admire the great thirteenth-century mosaics in the portal vaults. The angel on the Campanile bestows a special blessing in the milky light. Afternoon, we make our first foray into a museum, the Correr. Two works stand out for me – the *Pieta* of Tura and the Carpaccio of somewhat doubtful attribution, *Portrait of the Man in the Red Beret*. The *Pieta* so disturbing, an agonized Christ with a disbelieving Virgin holding him, turning away from his body but staring with intense focus at one still hand, as if desperately willing it back to life. An eternal plea. The Carpaccio is a small painting, the foreground taken up by the portrait of a wealthy merchant of most penetrating, steely, blue-eyed gaze, clad in a blue jacket beneath a coat of matching shade to his beret. He commands our attention.

We wander in a quite leisurely fashion around a museum that has not attracted many visitors this day. We think we will return. Dine very simply at A la Campagna, an albergo thankfully free of tourists. One large Italian family party joyously celebrating some anniversary.

MARCH 30: Quiet day orienteering. Go to the Rialto, stock up on fruit, marvelling at the size – and price – of the large white asparagus that is just beginning to appear.

In the course of these gentle forays, I noticed that Eric was taking a lot longer mastering the maps – always the simplest of tasks for him. I am eternally grateful that I did not resort to impatience, my normal response, but I remember thinking, He's suddenly getting older – or he's very preoccupied.

Bread, ham, purchased at the little shop near Corte Gregolini. Watching the owner wrapping produce with all the skill of a Japanese origami expert is a delight. Evening we dine at a popular restaurant, Da

Ivo, situated on a canal, and all the patrons exclaim with delight as the occasional gondola drifts past. We smile smugly, having flocks of them drifting past our dwelling.

MARCH 31: Easy day exploring all the calles and tiny campos within an easy radius. We notice the lion everywhere, slightly ferocious as becomes a patron beast. We discover some beautiful print shops, beautiful paper. Noted for later. Weather is good. We are content. Day nearly ruined by a meal at a restaurant near our apartment. Too awful to contemplate.

APRIL 1: The big foray to the Accademia. Bewildering assault by Titians, various related Bellinis, Carpaccio, Giorgione, Tintoretto ... on, on, Longhi, Bellotto, Guardi. We retire, defeated, having one or two favourites that can be drowned in later.

APRIL 2: The Doge's Palace in all its oppressive splendour ... Tintorettos, Titians, Veroneses, Tiepolos. We know they paint like huge angels, but so many of these paintings seem ordered up for the glory of Venice and the political requirements of the rulers of the day – they of absolute power. The Doge and his family lived in lofty grandeur. Way beneath them, the prisoners, the wicked who fell short of the Venetian interpretation of justice, languished, suffered, were tortured and died in tiny, icy cells.

Veronese's *Rape of Europa* brings a rare sensuality and lightness to the general gloom. Tintoretto's *Paradise,* sadly, under scaffolding ... Hieronymous Bosch, as usual, presenting an extraordinary revelation/nightmare right at the end of the museum. A near death experience in one of the paintings? Surely not!

In the evening, we attend a concert in a building opposite the side chapel of San Marco, which lifts our spirits to dizzying heights. This is a concert of Vivaldi, performed by the chamber orchestra Interpreti Veneziani. Having felt we never wanted to hear *The Four Seasons* again, we both feel we are hearing it for the first time. The players are all very young, all very pretty, and quite a few of them seem to be called Amadio.

APRIL 3: I am up early. A quarter to six. Drag on a bit of respectability, put lemon in hot water, proceed to desk. It is still, and the reflections in the canal perfect. Two bridges as clear in detail below as above. I contemplate picking up the phone. Instead, I listen to a miraculous stream of birdsong, which bounces off walls and then ascends. I am alone in Venice. Eric sleeps soundly.

There are no more diary entries.

I remember that day we went into a boutique and bought a handbag I had been coveting. On our way there, one of Venice's leashed dogs – a massive German shepherd – made a passing lunge at a Venetian cat, which fled in the opposite direction. But only for a moment. It returned at full gallop, scattering bystanders. Like many Venetian cats, it seemed to be the size of a small tiger; we regretted not being spectators at the imminent contest.

On the evening of Friday, April 3, we wandered through the Piazza, turned left along by the Canal, past the splendid sculpture of Casanova, up and over the bridge and into the Danieli. We intended booking a table for dinner the following week. We also went into Santa Maria della Pieta, Vivaldi's church, picked up a programme for forthcoming concerts, and finally made our destination for that evening, La Nuova Grotta, a restaurant down a calle off Riva degli Schiavoni, which I would never have located on my own. A lovely dinner, then a stroll back along the Grand Canal. That evening of April 3 was unbelievably lovely, with the moon casting reflections and making the waters gleam. We had just passed Casanova when Eric stopped and looked over towards Santa Maria della Salute. The moon had suffused one of the domes with light, and he looked at it intently for half a minute or more, not moving.

'That is so beautiful,' he said.

Santa Maria della Salute – the church dedicated to the Virgin and commissioned in 1630 in gratitude as the terrible plague receded. Literally, I discover later, St Mary of Health.

Eric was extraordinarily focused, very quiet, and we walked on in silence for a time, through a Piazza mercifully peaceful now, as it had been on the evening of the concert.

Not just in retrospect, but at the time, I was aware that we had finally unwound and that the next four weeks or so would be paradise. Paradise regained for Ruth and Eric. How truly lucky we seemed at that moment. Truly blessed.

He and I were right to come to Venice.

It is the early hours of the morning of April 4. I am vaguely aware of Eric in the bathroom at the basin. I am about to drift back to sleep but he has not returned to bed.

'Are you all right?'

'I seem to have a nose bleed. It's not bad. Go to sleep.'

I go back to sleep. When I wake later in the morning, he is in bed, on his back, with a handkerchief at his nose and a cold washer across the bridge.

'Hasn't it stopped?'

'No. Boring.'

I quickly make breakfast while he dresses in between wiping and staunching. He then lies on the sofa and I begin to feel niggles of anxiety. We have also run out of ice-blocks. I race to the farmacia near the Rialto and explain the situation with a mixture of mime and a few basic but, in these circumstances, fairly useless phrases. Having painstakingly struggled with the language for over three months, suddenly it is gone. I return with some help in the form of packs and dressings, which prove useless. It is still a steady, if slow, trickle. Finally –

'I think I'm going to need help.'

It is Saturday morning. This house has one permanent set of tenants – a family – none of whom I have seen, let alone met. There are travellers like us up above somewhere, now, doubtless, out exploring. I race back to the farmacia. All in attendance are serious and sympathetic and I am given the name of a medical group, which I am assured will be able to help.

I return, smiling at the figure on the sofa. I telephone. No answer. No recording machine either. I am really nervous now but have the sense to make one more call, leaving a message on Nicole's mobile to tell her I am having great difficulty getting a doctor and that Eric may have to go to Emergency.

I then run up the stairs to the first-floor apartment. The door is answered by a charming, brisk, late-middle-aged woman with not a word of English at her disposal. My mime and ten words convey the situation, and to the accompaniment of irritated male queries from the next room she disappears, returning with a bag of cotton balls. Finally, I persuade her that what I really need is the emergency number for an ambulance. This is graciously written, handed over with a tight smile, and the door politely but firmly closed in my face.

Trying to be brightly confident before my recumbent and, by now, very quiet spouse, I phone this number, which is of course not the ambulance but the police, who, thank God, not only speak English but are also able to make sense of my ramblings. I phone the correct number this time and order an ambulance. It is shortly after midday. We compose ourselves to wait.

I am concerned but not, I suppose, desperately worried at this stage – now that help is on the way. In my mind, ahead lies a trip to Emergency, some degree of plugging, then back here and early to bed, followed by a quiet Sunday. Then we will resume the idyll. Eric is making some attempt to read Linda La Plante in between wiping and sighing. I am looking out the window every few minutes, wondering where they will tie up. I had seen photos of a Venetian ambulance and crew because for some reason known only to himself, Eric, on one of his solitary forays this week, had photographed them in action. I am not at all entranced by life imitating art so swiftly.

There is a canal entrance to this building, but I should not think the doors have been opened for awhile. But where else ...? Every garbage barge, the police launch from the station at the corner of our tiny corte, all cause heart to leap ...

I make coffee and there is a pretence of eating something. One o'clock, two o'clock, and I am about to pick up the phone again when the bell rings and in come three characters straight out of an Italian movie, all fluoro jackets, energy and stethoscopes. Unambiguously theatrical. Their leader is a youthful Sophia Loren. She chews gum. There is one middle-aged man, and there is a young man who shuffles nervously and smiles reassuringly – the first action quite negating the second.

They banter among themselves in between questioning Eric loudly and slowly – they obviously think he is deaf. They are right, but both hearing aids *are* in place. The older man announces he will strap the nose, and my beloved is instantly transformed into a figure of fun with a bit of light plugging kept firmly in place by a strip of gauze. The gauze ends on top of his head, and when tied leaves him with two dangling rabbit ears. It seems we are now ready. He is placed in a primitive wheelchair and we journey forth into the alleys of Venice. If it were a sedan chair our journey may have had a touch of dignity. As it is, we push through the throngs, he stooped and dispirited, and I trying to behave as if we do this every day. We turn corner after corner, finally arriving at a small landing stage where the ambulance is moored. *This* is a first. The chair is lifted on, I follow – I cannot remember who drives – and very slowly we nose our way along narrow canals, edging close to gondolas, skilfully avoiding taxis, sliding around corners. The journey seems painfully slow. It is only when we eventually hit a relatively open stretch of water – the Grand Canal? – that the throttle is opened up. Thus does one get to hospital in Venice. I have no idea which direction we are headed in or where we are going, but at last we pull up alongside a building that was painted once by Bernardo Bellotto: *The Scuola di San Marco at San Giovanni e Paolo* – a painting we saw just three days earlier at the Accademia. It is now a hospital – Ospidale Civile San Giovanni e Paolo. None of this do I know yet.

All I do know is that Eric starts to faint and I am swiftly ordered away from the stretcher I have been leaning against for the journey. He is examined, has his blood pressure checked, recovers and is returned to the wheelchair. Our party proceeds from wharf to admitting room. He is admitted and we finally end up on the top floor of one wing of this ancient and beautiful, if crumbling, building.

There is a long wait, and while exploring the surroundings I am suddenly face to face with Nicole. I am astounded, having completely forgotten the phone call to her mobile. How she found us I am not sure, but we are now in very safe hands. Every step along the way from this moment will have her constantly on standby.

My guardian angel finally reveals herself.

Eric is very pale, and the wait for treatment is distressing. Not so distressing as the treatment itself, which is administered by a resident whose touch cannot be called gentle. Eric yells and I am ready to strike with handbag. Our worst moment is when this very handsome man, for whom I have developed a loathing, insists Eric stay overnight, as he will have lost quite a bit of blood. Eric is adamant that nothing will persuade him to stay, and I have to insist that he be discharged with myself taking full responsibility. The icy bargaining with the resident is conducted in French, a language we can attempt with some degree of success. We are very polite, though I do order him to take off his mask so I might hear what he is saying. Outside, Nicole is waiting for us.

Down to be discharged, and it is Nicole who is ushered in with Eric, to cope with the paperwork, while I sit in the waiting room, too tired to care whose husband they think he is. Adrenalin swiftly returns when the door opens and Nicole advises they are *insisting* on keeping him as he has collapsed again. The sight of my husband slumped and very weak is all the persuasion I need.

Back to the third floor, where, as a sweetener, we are offered a twin room – a huge concession in this public hospital – and I am able to assure him that we will be spending the night together. He is stoical. Nicole and I walk back to the apartment, and she painstakingly helps me to learn the route. I have no sense of direction, and the thought of returning to the hospital alone is terrifying; every signpost and landmark on the journey is gently hammered in by Nicole, while I do the laborious business of reversing in my mind as we walk.

I collect some night attire, toilet articles for us both, and set forth, literally whistling in the dark. Near the Rialto, I sit in a bar for a half hour and have a meal and a glass of wine, which are bad enough to match my mood. I head off again, but it all looks so different at night. I am unable to ask directions, so it is with a sense of immense relief that I do finally arrive at the last bridge and see the massive bulk of the hospital on the left of the campo.

I am shaking but triumphant – then manage to lose my way inside the hospital. Eventually, I rejoin Eric in our 'ensuite'. His relief is palpable. He has lived with my absence of any directional sense and probably feared we would never meet again. We are both desperate for this unpleasant interruption to our holiday to end.

He is ready for sleep and so am I. In the bathroom I discover that the tiny window looks directly onto the cemetery island, San Michele. It is strangely beautiful, but I do not dwell too long on the ghostly remains that inhabit it – Stravinsky, Diaghilev, Ezra Pound. Of course, this hospital and San Michele are ideally situated for mutual convenience – a convenience not necessarily pleasing to any patient looking out the window.

The next day is spent in relatively successful journeyings – sometimes accompanied by Nicole – between apartment and hospital. I decide to phone Sydney, thinking it foolish to conceal what I still hope is a somewhat minor hitch from family and close friends. All I speak to are concerned – very concerned – but it is important that I try to allay their fears. If I do not, I am fuelling my own, which I am keeping deeply buried.

I complete the last trip for the day and deliver treats and loving messages from home. We look ruefully at one another in our hospital room for two, each trying to reassure the other that this tiny nightmare will soon be over. I am suppressing the fact that he is too weak to go to the bathroom and that I am bringing the urine bottle to him as required – and what that may imply. All will be well! Why would he not be weak! Before we turn out the lights, Eric tells me of the vivid dream he had, just before waking with the nose bleed. It was a map of Venice, set out in tormenting and bewildering detail inches from his eyes. This alternated with a close-up of our address – 998 Corte Gregolini. He was obviously fearful of losing his way . . .

APRIL 6: I wake early – it is six o'clock. It is just light and I can hear him in the bathroom. He has taken himself there, obviously determined to prove a point. He returns and immediately falls back on his bed. I rush to him and he says, 'I'm numb down my side.' The next minute he is speaking an unknown language. It is not slurred; it is a very precise language. But it is a language from another planet.

I have never felt so frightened in my life. I am aware he has had a stroke – the implications are flooding every pore – I am calling out for assistance; I am ringing the bell; I am shouting, shouting; I am trying to tell the male nurse who finally appears that Eric has had a stroke; I am going mad; I do not know what to do; I do not know what will happen; he and I are alone in a slippery world; I am spinning out of control . . . I am going mad . . .

It only takes a moment for all systems to spring into action. Eric is surrounded by medical staff, and I pull back, allowing them to proceed. I am perfectly calm. Doctors are assessing his state and one of them tells me he will have to be moved immediately to 'Neurologica'. I nod and begin the business of packing up our belongings. Shortly, two female nurses arrive and Eric is transferred to a stretcher. They warn me that it is quite cold so I wrap my scarf around his head as we proceed to a lift. He is very calm, and on the way down he glances at one of the young women. To my surprise he winks at her – or is it a grimace, his face is twisted. I say, lightly, 'He always liked a pretty face,' which causes great merriment. We proceed jauntily out of the lift and into the cold morning air. He looks a little like Rudolf Valentino in my scarf; quite dashing if I ignore the twist on the right-hand side of his face. At last we get to Neurologica – there is a big board outside announcing it, and I think this will prove useful to me when next I try to find him. He is wheeled along one or two corridors – I am memorising as best I can – and ends up in another twin-bedded room; this time the other bed is occupied.

He is in need of another bottle, which fact is realised too late by the male nurse now in charge of him. This causes irritation, and his bedding is changed with a degree of force and grumbling that, fortunately, Eric is now beyond being bothered by. And they decide, of course, that he needs a catheter. As he is to undergo a number of tests and scans, I leave and return to the apartment. Coffee helps. I pick up the phone, first to Nicole and then to Anna, whose job it will be to pass on this melancholy development to all who need to know in Sydney – and in New Guinea, where Jonathan is. It is important for me to speak to our good friend John Rogers, a urologist/ surgeon. His phoning around Sydney to neurologists there and, time and again, to Eric's neurologists in Venice, is a source of great comfort. I am mostly kept completely informed. Anna and Jane are desperately anxious, but I am assured that one or other of the children will be arriving as soon as possible to lend support.

'Just hang on!'

Nicole has been busy shopping for me. We arrive at Eric's bedside with pyjamas, towels, face washers, new toilet articles. In Venice, patients have to be supplied with everything except bed linen, and the thin cotton towelling used only for the mopping up and cleaning of the patient when it is strictly necessary in the interests of hygiene. All other washing and sponging, feeding, nursing – apart from medical procedures and monitoring – are performed by the patient's relatives. This will be my job.

Eric is relieved to see us. He has a few words at

his command now – social words. What it must be like for him I cannot begin to imagine, but he is uncomplaining. I have the sense that his concern for me is perhaps stronger than his concern for himself. This is, after all, role reversal carried to extreme. He greets Nicole with warmth and appreciation, and desperately tries to make contact with, it must be said, a not particularly responsive nursing staff. Later, I realise that the hospital operates under extreme difficulties, is understaffed, and that the nursing shifts are punishing. Just now, I yearn for a greater degree of tenderness for him. I ache for them to respond. Their lack in this regard in no way dampens his desire to co-operate at all times, which I marvel at. The specialists who are attending him are charming and informative. It is a relief when they appear. They feel that the stroke is not a particularly serious one. I am shown x-rays and they do their best to reassure me. It is still a stroke though, and his right side is paralysed. What does concern them is the fact that his blood is not congealing – or coagulating as they say to me. The word will haunt me throughout this Venetian nightmare – 'No coagulation ... no coagulation ...' We start the process of trying to find out why.

'What medication is he on?'

I tell them Zocor and Cozaar, his blood-pressure medication. The packs are at his bedside. They examine them. They are *very* concerned about the blood, and I have to admit that from this moment my eyes are always straying to the bag under the bed, the one consistently visible sign of the problem.

'He could have been poisoned,' they say, brightly.

I am aghast. What are we talking about here? Strychnine? Arsenic? Ant-Rid?

They enjoy this moment.

'No! No! No! – Food! What restaurants have you been to?'

I go back over the past few days, but we are not making much progress.

I mention that, as a sufferer from sinusitis, he had squirted a saline solution into his nostrils the night before the nose bleed. And that, as he had run out of the pharmaceutical solution, he had concocted his own, using bottled water that was aerated. This interests them more. I also mention that at the beginning of the year he suffered a minor injury to his head that bled profusely, perhaps too profusely. They nod, make a note, and prepare to leave – again assuring me that the stroke is not a major one.

I return to his bedside. The man who occupies the other bed is up and wandering about in his dressing gown. He is enormously helpful in explaining hospital procedures, and his English is perfect. He becomes my interpreter when Nicole is absent, and his obvious concern for our situation is touching.

I stay for a time and then return to the apartment. Nicole is working in the other apartments. The owner lives on the second floor, and washing and ironing is done there by Nicole. She is to add extra laundry for me over the weeks, particularly as my children arrive and bunk down. There is also a laundromat around the corner. We had already availed ourselves of their services – take your washing, put it in the machine, come back, get it out. Just the usual, I imagine. Over the weeks, the two women who run this will take my washing, do it for me, fold it. They turn to me the instant I enter their tiny shop, ignoring others – pause at the ironing board, exchange glances, murmur their concerns. I have become a celebrity by virtue of an ill husband.

'On holidays, too. It is very terrible!'

Back to the hospital.

We are both being stupidly cheerful. What else? No alternative.

Back to the apartment.

I am surprised how well I sleep.

APRIL 7: A beautiful day as I push through the tourists. There are two kinds of Venetian. The indolent stroller who blocks the path with sublime confidence, and the committed walker whose pace is Olympian. Already, I am metamorphosing into the second. I stride through the calles. My pace is fast. I become expert in avoiding knots of people who suddenly materialize in front of me. They melt away for me, as they do for Venetians.

I pick up a few necessary items at the supermarket on the way, then fruit at the shop near the hospital. The fruit, the tomatoes, all vegetables, are wonderful. The man who serves me recognizes me now. We banter a little. Nothing has changed much in the hospital room. Eric's bed is against the wall. I sit on the other side, making the mandatory, surreptitious check of the bag at the side of the bed. I do not like what I see. The doctors come and go. They ask me to wait. Nicole pops in on her way to the apartments. As I am seeing her out she suddenly begins to cry, and I find *I* am comforting *her,* one arm around her shoulders.

'Don't ... don't, it's all right!'

'Mrs Phillips, it's so awful! He's on his holiday!'

'We'll be all right. Don't worry.'

Keep smiling ... keep smiling ... keep smiling ...

I return to the room and wait. He sleeps. Leads and tubes everywhere, blood dripping in, dripping out ... Late in the morning, a trio of neurologists enters the room, one older and obviously senior. They carry reports, x-rays.

The older man asks me to accompany him. Along more corridors, round corners, and we are in his office. He is the Primario of the Neurology section of the hospital. He speaks to me for some minutes, expressing his concern at the 'non-coagulation of the blood ...' He informs me that he must send Eric to Intensive Care immediately. He is an extremely kind man, very serious, as he explains the ramifications of Eric's bewildering state. The blood problem is mysterious ...

His words are gentle, but there is a subtext here. I am good at subtexts. I cut through the words ...

'Doctor, are you telling me that my husband's condition could be fatal?'

I do not believe I am saying these words. Maybe I am not. I am acutely aware of grave eyes locked into mine.

'Yes.'

There, he has said it. I must have asked the question.

I do not know how long we sit there. It does not matter. Nothing matters.

After awhile, my next sentence oozes out –

'My children should all fly over?'

'Yes. In my opinion. I am very sorry.'

What a bastard of a job you've got, Doctor.

I am back in Eric's room. Lunch is being served. His companion is sitting quietly on the side of his bed eating. The sides of Eric's bed are up. He must have some secret knowledge. He is turned away from me facing the wall, his good arm flung over the side. He is in a foetal position. One of the few times on this whole journey that I witness any despair. Very quickly, there are nurses and wardsmen crowding around and they wheel him out. I begin to gather up his things, as Nicole materializes – of course – and helps me. I had not realised there was so much ...

We take our leave of his companion, now resting on the bed. He rises.

'I hope everything will go well with your husband.'

I thank him. Nicole and I arrange to meet at Intensive Care around six o'clock.

That afternoon I go inside San Marco for the very first time. Not through the great front doors under the four horsemen, but into the side chapel, where one or two people are praying. I sit near the front, and my eyes are on the icon to the right of the altar. The Virgin's eyes gaze out, slightly to the left of mine; the child she holds in an awkward, upright position is an antique baby. I stare at them. I do not want to leave. I may stay here forever ...

Later, I stride through the Piazza. The stupid strings, decked out in white tuxedos, are playing Lehar of all things. I stand still, with tears streaming down my face, oblivious of the nervous glances cast my way. How in God's name did all this happen? What am I doing? Why am I here?

Eric and I had flown out of Sydney a lifetime ago. As far as I knew, he was completely healthy. He had been working six days a week, leaving home every morning at six and walking a couple of kilometres before breakfast.

Ten days after arriving in Venice, my husband is in Intensive Care. Someone has told me he is dying and no one seems to know why. I am in the middle of a nightmare, but I cannot wake up. I am not going to wake up ...

Why Venice? What could have possessed us?

Throughout 1997, through the hustle and the bustle and the comings and the goings, the highs, the excitements; the on-again off-again ramifications of establishing another gallery in which Eric was actively involved – the one thing that kept us sane and afloat was a small beacon glowing softly at year's end, our holiday! As we drew nearer and the beacon shone clearer, we were like children about to enter the lolly shop. He and I were off to New York.

Eric had been to New York many times – first, when he was working for AWA, and in later years, after we had started our business, travelling there for framing and print conventions. We had even managed to be there together once or twice – purely, deliciously, sinfully, on a holiday.

We both loved New York, and as our friend John McKellar would be there, we vowed to visit both him and the city the minute I was free of *Vita and Virginia* and the book tour. We would have Christmas at home and fly out on Boxing Day. Eric was determined that I should see New York in winter.

We decided to spend at least three weeks there, possibly more. We would stay, as usual, at the Wyndham, right opposite the Plaza, and we would certainly treat ourselves to one meal, or at the very least, a pre-dinner drink across the street. Oh yes! One cannot visit New York at Christmas and miss the Plaza's decorations, my dear!

Or *any* of New York's decorations – or the icy cold outside and the warmth inside, or the shopping, or the Metropolitan, or the MOMA, or the Guggenheim, or the Frick, or the Pierpont Morgan Library, or the book shops, or New Year's Eve …

It seemed, as 1997 hurtled away, the perfect start to the New Year. Would I find it necessary to treat myself to a new coat, I wondered? A trunk-load of books perhaps? Warm thoughts like this flickered away happily beneath the demands of that busiest year of my life.

I hope they were flickering in Eric's mind that September when pleurisy struck him. It happened when I was on tour, and he managed to keep the extent of his illness from me. As usual, he rarely took any time off, but on one occasion he had to call for medical help in the middle of the night. This I only discovered well after the event.

Throughout our marriage Eric had barely had a

day's illness. Flu mostly stayed away from him, any cold behaved itself. He was an extremely healthy man, his one visit to hospital during our marriage being for a routine prostate operation, which I seem to remember put him in a very bad mood. He was not a good patient for the few hours that he ever admitted to being one. Once the pleurisy passed, little mention was made of it.

Then, just before 1997 ended, the Sydney Theatre Company proposed a return season of the highly successful *Vita and Virginia.* It was scheduled for the end of January at the Opera House.

A major spanner had been thrown into the works.

'Your decision.'

This was his response to my agonizing over whether or not to accept – as it always was where my professional activities were concerned. We were both delighted by the audience response to *Vita and Virginia.* He loved this play and, I heard later, felt it to be my best role. So I made my decision.

With the ABC by now wanting an audio of 'the book', our first available date to leave would be the end of March. We blocked April/May out of our diaries and re-thought our destination. John no longer in New York in April, that city's interest diminished somewhat. Our minds were open. In the middle of the year, I would be rehearsing Edward Albee's *A Delicate Balance,* so the timing, which was now sacrosanct, would work very nicely.

One evening, when we were sitting on the side verandah waiting for the news … he sipping his vodka … I musing … suddenly, like a bolt from the blue, a message from on high, Moses bringing down the tablet …

'Venice! Venice! We should go to Venice!'

He looked up.

'Venice?'

'Yes! Yes! Venice!'

He chuckled.

'You're right! That's it! We'll go to Venice!'

So, why *Venice*?

I am still not sure. Perhaps because Venice has a fascinating and unique history that pleaded for greater research. As we dipped into the odd book, we swiftly became hooked.

Here was a city that had only come into being

because a community of people moved sideways out of the path of some rapidly approaching, plundering, extremely barbaric hordes. How clever those first Venetians were, simply stepping to one side. The hordes thus missed them and had to continue south for their fun. Then, upon finding that at the coast, after their shrewd two-step, they were in decidedly marshy country, the cunning, embryonic Venetians simply put their dwellings on stilts.

The small, marshy community was the source of what was to become a great maritime and mercantile city. As it grew, Venice was ideally placed to take full advantage of the newly opening trade routes. A city for merchants, in other words. A city, too, for all who made their living from the sea, for mariners who flocked in and out, bringing their own marvellous fables to add to Venice's own. A city, above all, for the adventurous and curious, like Marco Polo, who travelled forth on sea and land to find out what was around the corner, or, like Galileo, what was way, way up and beyond.

Over the centuries, Venice became the prosperous city, the clever city, the Serene City – serene, presumably, because everything worked so sweetly for her. Ultimately, too, the city of power – which meant that great buildings were erected, not only for those wealthy merchants and their governors to work and live in, but also to praise God for all his blessings and to thank him with yet another grand church whenever plague, a not infrequent visitor, released its terrible grip. And those great buildings and churches needed to be filled with beautiful artworks. Venice eventually provided these herself.

All this was reason enough for us.

There was more, of course. The indefinable quality of any great city, which can be lumped under the general heading Spirit of Place. What is Venice's? If one is to believe all the words written, the paintings executed, the films produced, that 'spirit' would seem to be romantic. Romantic and sensuous and sensual. The city created for love; city of Casanova, the greatest lover of all if his own testimony is to be believed. Thrown into prison when his excesses got out of hand. Thrown into prison – and then allowed to escape. Escape in Venice, if one is clever enough at disappearing down side passages and has many friends, means vanishing. What stories there are of Casanova, of his amours. What endurance. The romance of a gondola nosing quietly, secretly, to some deserted landing spot, the beautiful masked passenger disguised as a man revealing herself at last, after plunging the waiting lover into despair. The trickery of love acted out with an instinct, surely, for the possibility that one day this pretty play will end up on canvas, in a sculpture, or in someone's film.

Being escorted to the place of love by the one who bestowed his name on all would-be imitators, where refreshment awaits in a setting of exquisite charm, and where the persuasive game to follow will be swift and irresistible. Or so I, also a romantic, insist on believing. And that the beloved could be a beautiful and demure nun weighed not at all in the scheme of things.

Love and excess everywhere! A convent where the attending friar will take *his* pleasures among the sweet-faced nuns. And ultimately pay quite a price. But who has asked the nuns what *their* views were? Perhaps, despite their high and solemn vows, their accommodation of the wicked friar was not entirely without a degree of acquiescence. Many of them had come from the aristocracy – no strangers themselves to unacceptable behaviour. Who knows? We all guess. But the secrecy of Venice, the trickiness of Venice – two faces presented to the world, one romantic and seductive, the other, concealed always by a mask, licentious, libidinous and cruel – this, too, is part of Venice's spirit of place.

Chiaroscuro. The word seems invented for her. Clear and dark. Subtle changes of light wherever you look; what you think you see is not what you get; watery concealment ... sometimes, too, concealment of the most horrible with the utterly poetic. What other city would name the bridge over which so many shuffled to their doom the Bridge of Sighs? The name colours our perception of the reality, softening the horror.

What other city, tell me, made the mask an art form? And still does.

While we were perusing and pondering these impressions of other travellers, references to Venice began to appear everywhere – on television and in newspaper articles, radio interviews, advertising. It seemed a beneficent fate was approving our change of direction. The film *Wings of the Dove,* based on the Henry James novel, opened to a rapturous reception; many people we knew had recently returned from Venice; and Venetian paintings and posters started to appear everywhere, as if by magic.

We had both been, separately, to Venice in the fifties and been bewitched. In my diary of the European journey of that time it is the only entry that ends, rather grandiosely, 'Yes, one will return ...'

SUMMER 1953: Venice, which of course preceded Padua, regrettably, we could only give a cursory glance to. A trip along the Grand Canal by ferry (so much cheaper than gondola if slightly less romantic) passing under the famed Rialto. This is the most fascinating city I have seen – the Byzantine influence most apparent – a tiny side canal the most intriguing thing imaginable. How the buildings seem to *grow* out of the water. And the quaint garb of the gondoliers, with the beribboned straw hats, adds to the impression of unreality that Venice gives on all sides. St Mark's Square makes departure from Venice agony. A return is imperative, and it is only a half-thought promise to oneself that return will be made that makes departure possible. The swirling, fluttering, strutting pigeons, the grace of the Doge's Palace, the impossibility that is the Cathedral, the clock, the people, all cast their irresistible spell, and, yes, one *will* return ...

Who would dare go against such breathless conviction?

Thus were we pulled inexorably towards that 'abhorrent, green slippery city', as D. H. Lawrence would have it. Eric extracted all relevant information from the Internet, and gradually the 'Venice' file began to outstrip all others. Friends delivered books and restaurant guides, and Ron Blair, who had spent three months in Venice in a writer's studio, gave us enough material to gain a Master's on the city. Eric devoured more of the information than I did, but that has usually been our way – he researching, planning, I pottering along happily behind, always more at home with the broad picture than the detail, the atmosphere, the spirit of place, preferring to be *drenched* by it all.

We hurried to see *Wings of the Dove,* concentrating far more on the exquisitely filmed scenes of Venice than the subtleties of Henry James.

My daughter Anna saw the film, too; said to a friend afterwards,

'I have to go to Venice.' Within weeks she was handing over her youngest child to be looked after.

Wish granted.

And, once the decision was made, the planning became more and more adventurous. It was developing into one of our better journeys. After Venice, a few days in Barcelona, and then a week or so with dear friends, Gully and Tim Cavanough, in their house in Majorca. They spend six months of every year in Sydney and six months in Majorca. Our timing matched theirs perfectly. They would be in Majorca in April/May, and we were urged to take as much time as we could. Their village would be ready and waiting. Not just a journey then, but the holiday of a lifetime.

So it seemed ...

The return season of *Vita and Virginia* in 1998 ran through the great Mardi Gras festival in Sydney, that extraordinary celebration of all things gay and extravagant. That time when Sydney explodes with tourists and dollars and there is a huge parade, watched by thousands, that causes some division within the city – on the one hand, the keeper of the city's morals, Fred Nile and his followers, praying for rain to mar the event, on the other everyone joyously and rudely ignoring him. The festival is preceded by a concert to publicise all the events – straight and gay – that will be happening throughout Sydney at the time. Someone had the bright idea that Jennifer Hagan and I should appear at this concert. It coincided with the second night of our run, and the Sydney Theatre Company ordered a vintage Rolls to transport Vita Sackville-West and Virginia Woolf in style to the State Theatre – and then forgot to send a photographer to record the scene. Our dresser kindly took snaps. The two literary ladies walked onto the stage, had a reception that all but lifted the roof off the State, and instead of quitting while in front, Jenny and I performed a somewhat inept, brief sketch publicising our play, thus ruining the moment. The whole concert was called *The Stars Come Out,* which title, in my usual vague way, I only discovered after the event. Ah well ... it added an extra mystique to our season, perhaps.

I could not believe what fate had thrown at me over the past year. Up, up, to dizzying heights – *Vita and Virginia* and *A Little Night Music*; a successful book launch; 1998 providing a play I was eager to tackle, Edward Albee's *A Delicate Balance*; a commercial run of *A Little Night Music*; a great holiday just around the corner; and, most surprising of all, discovering I was one of a hundred people in the country chosen as National Living Treasures. It was a dangerously high crest. I was torn between writing and acting – was quite unsure what I wanted to do. I could, it seemed, head off in any direction. Or stop altogether. Crossroads.

'There's only one thing I know with absolute certainty. When I get to Venice, I will know!'

My name might have been Icarus.

It is six o'clock. Nicole has collected me from Corte Gregolini. We have made our way through the Venetian streets and I am astounded at how many people know her. She is constantly waving and greeting, stopping for a short time. I am glad of the distractions.

'Ciao, Nicole.'

'Ciao.'

Earlier, I had phoned Sydney. Shocked. But Jonathan will be flying over with Jane. Anna will take a day or two longer to organize four children.

'You're in our thoughts! We're with you ...'

Everyone I speak to.

'I'm lighting candles,' say some.

Everyone in a state of disbelief ...

We arrive at Intensive Care, me trying to etch the direction onto my brain. On the way, through the lovely courtyards with their neglected and heartbreakingly beautiful gardens, we have passed many, many cats. Some are eating. Some are sleeping. Others watch. I am surprised to see one actually inside the Intensive Care building. I become used to him – pale ginger. He occupies a niche. I miss him if he is not there.

We go up to the first floor. There is a small waiting room with a television set, which is not turned on. Two anxious elderly people waiting quietly and patiently. One or two others sitting outside on the chairs lining the wall. We join them, leaving our umbrellas neatly stacked – it has been raining. There is a closed door leading into the Intensive Care ward through which doctors, nurses, occasionally pass. Nicole tells me a doctor will open the door at some time to give information. Nicole has already announced our arrival through an intercom.

And we wait.

The elderly couple is summoned. Conversation ensues. They quietly leave. They have not seen their loved one.

Others go to the intercom and try to get information. It is obvious that any human presence is strictly rationed.

One hour passes. Two. I can feel my anger rising. We did, after all, arrive at the appointed time.

Some people are admitted into the inner sanctum.

I explode and demand that Nicole get us some satisfaction. Nervously, she addresses the intercom again. I tell her these meek Venetians are too compliant by half.

'You must be patient, Mrs Phillips! They will let us in when they are able.'

After three hours a doctor opens the door fractionally and we have our conversation. Nicole translates. I am not to be allowed to see him tonight. He is 'critical', puncture pinholes throughout the gastro-intestinal tract, liver affected, no coagulation, no coagulation, no coagulation ... Fighting every emotion at once, I ask whether it is worthwhile my children flying half way across the world to see their father.

'Will he still be alive on Thursday evening?' Pushing the sarcasm down ...

I am shaking but very controlled. She gives me a bright, cool smile –

'Cross fingers your husband will still be alive!'

Now rage takes over. Nicole's hand is on my arm.

'Mrs Phillips, Mrs Phillips, don't be upset, don't be upset. You must stay calm. Cross fingers in

Venice means, yes he *will* be alive. It's a message of good luck.'

I am not convinced, but we leave. I cannot accept that I am unable to see him tonight. We are to return at the same time tomorrow.

Nicole leaves me after five minutes' walk, and I retrace the journey to the apartment. I am getting very good at it now, although my way *is* the long way. Stick with what you know. No emotion left. Venice looks beautiful, as ever. Up and over the bridges. It is no longer raining, but the wet pavements throw reflections. Water on all sides. It feels soothing.

I go into A la Campagna, the albergo Eric and I had found, and have a quick meal and a small jug of wine. Grilled fish – and green peas to which I have become addicted. I think they are tinned, but I cannot get enough of them. They mash beautifully. Nursery food. I pay the bill. The young manager recognizes me now. Gives me a quiet corner. Knows that on my first visits I was accompanied.

Arriving at the apartment I find I cannot open the door. The key has always been a little temperamental, and tonight it is not going to co-operate at all. I struggle, am plunged into darkness, go back to the street door, re-activate the light ... If it does not work this time, I tell myself, it is straight into the canal. The devil within the key knows I mean business and the lock turns smoothly. I go inside and pick up the phone.

It is a beautiful day when I open the shutters next morning. The sounds rush in, the bells are chiming, there is bustle on the canal, the gondoliers are starting up their singing, which has by now definitely lost its charm. If I escape from Venice I never wish to hear *Santa Lucia* or *Come Back to Sorrento* again. Piano accordians are off the list, too. Over at the hotel it is changeover day for the tourists – the taxis are already loading up. Garbage barges nose along, and there is delivery of flour, sugar, stacked laundry. These craft tie up and someone is waiting to transport the loads on wheels – wheels that are moved by human sweat. Venice is medieval. Everything is pushed and pulled. Garbage is placed out at night in plastic shopping bags. You see the bags outside all the doors. It is collected, tossed onto a cart and then pushed to the nearest landing. In our tiny corte, the top-floor residents of the adjacent building lower a supermarket bag of garbage every night except Saturday – no collection on the Sabbath. It hangs just above ground level, dangling jauntily. Outside the windows, four storeys up, the washing dries. There is always a lot of washing, which hangs on an intricate pulley system of lines. Down below, adolescent boys kick soccer balls around the corte. They make a deal of work for whoever manipulates the lines above them. They are polite boys and never kick the ball as I am crossing.

I buy provisions, write cards, visit my Madonna, sitting quietly – try to fill in the hours till evening. The weather has gone through four seasons today, and this will be the pattern for the rest of April – T. S. Eliot's 'cruellest month'. To go forth without an umbrella invites disaster.

I cannot wait for six o'clock. I dread six o'clock.

Nicole and I are seated along the wall, wet umbrellas drying. Her very presence is calming. With her there I feel I can face what is ahead. It will be dealt with. A doctor emerges en route elsewhere when a phone sounds in the waiting room. He answers it, and to my astonishment asks for 'Signora Phillips'.

I cannot believe I am talking to Jonathan, who has somehow managed to find me in a waiting room in the middle of a vast hospital in Venice! He sends words of encouragement and gives me his arrival time. Jane will be with him. Nicole has already announced firmly that she will be meeting them at the airport. It is unbelievably wonderful to hear from him.

Then, I am called. I enter Intensive Care. One or two people intent on screens; someone wanders past. It is quiet. I am given plastic gear – overshoes, head cover, gown …

'Cinque … cinque …'

I presume we are talking minutes. I go through the door.

He lies on a catafalque. He is majestic, what is left of him. Intravenous leads carrying blood, nourishment. Machines blipping, lights. I stand still, as if waiting for something. He turns his head and sees my plastic-covered form …

A great shout echoes through Intensive Care – a clarion call to rock the walls of Jericho.

'I KNOW *YOU*!' is the cry. 'I LOVE *YOU*!'

I go to him and can barely get at him. But do … There are the beginnings of a beard as I touch his face. We are content to be silent. I cannot begin to imagine what these hours since we last saw one another must have been like for him. No knowledge of the language, he could have been in a space capsule hurtling towards another planet. Kidnapped by aliens. No communication whatever for over thirty hours. I only hope someone touched him occasionally.

I am leaning over the cot, and after a time he says, with great clarity –

'It was so beautiful! I was so happy!'

As I try to digest this – and he says it with all the urgency he can muster – his face is, if I say suffused with a kind of joy, who is going to believe me, but I say it anyway.

I report.

I am looking at him, astonished, and not listening carefully enough to his next words, but I hear him say, 'She …' 'She,' he says, more than once. 'She …'

What follows, I simply do not hear, I am too involved in the moment –

'She … She …'

– and I miss it! Involved, as ever, in the big picture, the detail escapes me. To my continuing regret …

Five minutes have more than passed. I am frightened of tiring him, so I say good-bye and tell him I shall be back with Jane and Jonathan.

Jane and Jonathan arrived in Venice in the middle of the afternoon of April 9, escorted by Nicole. She left us together and we arranged to meet later at Intensive Care. It seemed an eternity since I had seen them. It was. They stacked their baggage, which included a sleeping bag, and we went out for coffee and took Jane to the Piazza. Then it was time for us to head towards the hospital. We walked along my route, and they marvelled at the number of tourists everywhere. We slipped into one of the churches on our way – just to get a glimpse of paintings and sculptures, a taste of the Venice that is Venice. But there was something else throbbing away inside them – the paintings irrelevant.

How to prepare them for what they would so soon see? I said the words but knew they were not going to make any difference. The words were just words. Useless things in the face of their coming encounter.

We were admitted into Intensive Care as a family, but we had decided that I should see him first, and then it would be their turn. So I left them covering themselves in plastic and went to him. The amount of plastic protection I was wearing this time was somewhat less than on my first visit – there did not seem to be any standardization. I suspected it depended on whoever was supervising the activity.

His relief and delight at my approach were heartbreaking. I leaned on the side of his bed. Did we speak? I cannot really remember. I read him a card of love and encouragement from Anna. Nothing else. But then, somehow, I found myself singing to him. Crooning away softly and singing, of all things, a twenties ballad I had not thought of in decades.

If You Were the Only Girl in the World – on, on I went through the lyric ...

> If you were the only boy in the world
> And I were the only girl
> Nothing else would matter in the world today
> We would go on living in the same old way
> A garden of Eden just made for two
> With nothing to mar our joy ...

And then he was singing with me.

There we are, Ruth and Eric, arm in arm, doing a dance step along a beach somewhere – he in natty straw boater, I all innocent smile and floating sash. What fun! Then it dawns on me ...

'My darling, you're singing in tune! It's a miracle!'

He gave me his twisted grin and the ghost of a laugh struggled out.

'And in the right key ... how did you manage that? First time in forty years!'

I could see the others waiting and watching and called them in. I left them.

How can they cope. Their father is wrecked, beached, washed in by the tide, helpless, entangled in seaweed and shells, and he is crying.

This is the worst moment of their lives. Jonathan, who has been in other countries for most of his working life, has been used to lightning trips home, the charged warmth of welcome – excitement, feast days. We visited him when he was flying out into the North Sea from Aberdeen, and it was holiday time for the three of us. Perhaps Jonathan has always brought that sense of recreation with him. And his father was constantly buoyant in his presence. Jane? Jane has worked with him for many years in an office just a short walk down a hallway from *his* office. In some ways she saw more of him than I did. She was the last one to see him before he shut the door on work. When he was off on a magical journey. When he was very, very happy.

We leave him, and they are soon walking along the broad, marble-tiled hallway that leads to the outside world. I walk behind them, watching. Their heads are bowed and soon they are walking with their arms around one another. They are wounded.

We head into the evening light, by now Jonathan ahead with his thoughts – which are murderous – Jane and I walking in silence. I take them to my albergo where we dine simply, I wolfing the green peas. We are determined on a long consultation the next day with Intensive Care staff, neurologists and anyone else who can throw some light on Eric's parlous state. Anna is due to arrive on Saturday. Her card to me is in my new shoulder bag, my one Venetian purchase. I have the card still. I pay the young manager, who had politely noticed he was now seating three.

In our apartment for two, three are now bedding down. We have made arrangements with Nicole to meet at the hospital in the morning, when our quest for information will begin. Jonathan unrolls a sleeping bag; Jane and I will share the bed. They have lighter moments, looking out the windows up and down the sparkling canals, listening to night sounds . . . We go to bed at last. It is indescribably wonderful to have them round me.

The next day, Friday, we start pushing for information. After Nicole has started the process with Intensive Care, we are told to wait, and we wave her good-bye. Jonathan has a notebook at the ready and it is not too long before we are seated in the office of someone designated the Primario of Internal Medicine. Internal Medicine is in the opposite wing and up a floor from Intensive Care. This man is Dr Gabriele Bittolo Bon. He is urbane, handsome, confident, and exudes an optimistic approach to life in general and medical problems in particular, which will keep us going for the rest of our stay. He is one of the loveliest men I have ever met.

He begins a discussion with the doctor from Intensive Care, which, being in Italian, sounds suspiciously like a confrontation that can only end with pistols at dawn. We pick up enough to know that Intensive Care do not in the least wish to release their patient. It is my belief that the Primario is never bested. Intensive Care retires defeated. I have been looking around his room with its blown-up photographs of sea and dolphins and family and frolicking, together with some art pieces and books. In this hospital, of course, it is not a grand room, but it is welcoming. Finally, he turns to us. He tells us that Eric has had many scans and x-rays, that – as we knew – he has this blood condition which, in his case, is dangerous and unpredictable, that his stroke is manageable, that there is a spot on his lung. The blood condition can be triggered by infection or trauma, such as an accident of some kind, and the Primario is opting for infection because of the spot on the lung, which he takes to be pneumonia. Eric will be fed antibiotics intravenously. He is not fit to travel, but the aim will be to get him to a level of stability where travel *can* be contemplated. With the infection cleared, the blood condition should improve. In the meantime, the Primario feels it is imperative for Eric to have his family around him, and has taken the step of having him moved to Internal Medicine. The Primario's smile indicates that it was a good fight and one that it is only proper for him to have won.

'After all,' he says, smiling broadly, 'he is just a short trolley journey from Intensive Care!'

He has decided to place Eric in a twin-bedded

room, which means that I shall be able to sleep there every night. This is an extraordinary and generous gesture and one that is seldom granted to Italians, who sit up all night in waiting rooms and face the next day exhausted and stiff and remain there as long as there is danger. A weight has been lifted. The next time we see Eric he will be in a room.

Dr Bittolo Bon's English is not good, but it is good enough for those of us who are woefully lacking in his language. We shake hands, and for the first time since Monday morning I feel a little hopeful.

We are by now in touch with the Consulate in Rome. No foreign representation in Venice is another good reason for not falling ill here. In Sydney, a friend has already spoken to Foreign Affairs advising of our plight, and the Consul, Charles Farrugia, will be calling on us over Easter. We have spoken to him and been introduced, over the phone, to the Vice-consul, Teraseta Iglesius, and her assistant, Rita Trivellioni, who is to assume a major role in the forthcoming dramas. Teraseta and Rita will prove two lifelines to sanity. Our little world is broadening.

I take my two to a pleasant lunch. A pattern

begins to emerge. I will insist over the coming weeks that we resolutely allow ourselves an hour for lunch and for unwinding. This is my wisest decision, perhaps, and allows us to maintain the strengths that are vital for survival all round. We return to the hospital, I relieved to leave it to them to find Internal Medicine through the maze of this place. By our last day here, I am very familiar and cocky, but now it is still a nightmare. After all, Eric will have entered his fifth department in this hospital.

On the ground floor is a bar, which will prove to be life-saving. It sells bottled water, croissants (not so good), coffee (excellent), biscuits, yogurts – extras, in other words. I will be slipping in there often for a tiny plastic cup of espresso. It is near a telephone, which eventually I am able to master.

Internal Medicine is entered by way of a lift opening off an outside laneway. The entry is alongside the kitchen, where, behind thick plastic curtains, steaming cauldrons turn out the quite acceptable meals that feed this large community. Sometimes the place seems like a foretaste of Dante's *Inferno,* all shouts and clouds of steam and bangings and scourings, with fearsome characters in Wellington boots sweeping and scrubbing with immense brooms.

On Eric's floor, the third, we make enquiries, are identified as the Australians and questioned, yet again, as to medication and any event that may or may not have precipitated his disaster. Unnecessary, in my view, but presumably essential for the charming and elegant woman, Dr Mariateresa Busetto, who is in charge on this floor. I go through it once more – Zocor ... Cozaar ... nasal douche ... the excessive bleeding from the minor wound. It is all noted down.

He is ready for our visit and we go into the room with its two beds. Mine is the one near the window, looking across the inner garden to the other wing – Intensive Care, where if necessary he can be rushed, across and down a floor. He is still festooned with leads carrying blood and antibiotic and whatever else needs to drip in; and the bag beneath the bed is visible (already Jane and Jonathan are doing surreptitious checking). Now, though, he can begin to eat again.

There is a small cupboard, the bedside tables, and the door to a bathroom that I shall be sharing with a very elderly lady, whose stockings frequently hang there to dry and where still-to-be-discovered horrors will await me. Thank God there is a hand basin in the room.

It is pleasant enough. He has greeted us with the cheery 'Halloo' – rather like a hunting cry – that will be his call whenever he is not too ill for greeting. We take it in turns to sit on the chair, wander about, make a note of what is needed in the room. We tell him the consul will be calling, which delights him; we give him news from home. We have access to him twenty-four hours a day, and the Primario is now in charge. We can get to the Primario pretty often, too. We are blessed. I tell him I will not be staying this first night – there is too much to organize – but I shall be staying every night after that. I will see him again tonight and bed him down, which means sponging and soothing. Three trips to Ospidale Civile this Friday, but how wonderful to see him in a room, how wonderful to know we do not have to be separated. Feels like paradise.

On Saturday, Anna will be arriving. Jonathan, who knows his way around Venice, will go to the airport to meet her. One more reunion, and I stoutly refuse to linger on the reason that will have our family together as a family for the first time in over twenty years – though not quite together.

One of us has to be sure to be with him at meal times as his paralysed right arm and all the tubes make it very difficult, if not impossible, for him to feed himself. It all works out. Food, from this moment, is of paramount importance to him. He does not lose his appetite and I am never sure whether he is resolutely going through the business of eating simply to stay alive or whether there is genuine enjoyment in it for him. A little of each, probably.

When Anna received my phone call on the Wednesday, she took the train to Sydney to arrange matters there, returned home and organized her family, and then drove to Sydney with her husband, John, on the Friday. He and Lisa put her on the plane. One of the last to speak to Anna was John Rogers, who had been talking to specialists in Sydney and in Venice. He needed to say something ...

'Anna, I should tell you, you must prepare yourself for the fact that Eric may have died before you get there. I'm so sorry.'

With this news accompanying her, Anna flew to Bangkok, changed planes, flew to Rome, and boarded the plane for Venice with the heaviest of hearts. As she was nearing the terminal in Venice she could see Jonathan waiting. His demeanour, glimpsed at a distance, convinced her that her father had indeed died; she approached with dread.

Unexpectedly given some very welcome news, Anna arrived at Corte Gregolini, if not smiling, at least relieved to a point approaching cheerfulness. We were all infected briefly. It was quite delightful.

She saw him that evening. Another joyous reunion, more tears ...

Eric's greeting next day when she arrived at the hospital was somewhat different.

'What are *you* doing here?' were his first words. He was cross now, having just realized that three extra plane fares were involved. He groaned considerably as he made rapid mental calculations – dollars bleeding away in all directions. We told him airily to pay no attention whatever. Everything had been taken care of.

'Absolutely nothing to worry about!' we said.

'Cross our hearts and hope to die!'

Life in Venice settled swiftly into a routine. My absence at night at the hospital meant that an apartment designed to take two could be stretched to take the four of us – just. Anna and Jane shared the bed, Jonathan unrolled his sleeping bag every night. I returned for breakfast in the morning.

Marketing was done, laundry dropped around the corner – clothing only, everything else was whipped away by Nicole and returned pressed and neatly folded; we reminded ourselves to put the supermarket bag of garbage out every night; visits to the hospital were shared; interviews as to Eric's current state, and the prognosis, undertaken by all four of us, notebooks at hand.

And our lunches continued to soothe and strengthen. Sometimes we barely spoke. Sometimes we could even pretend we were on a holiday – for a minute or two ...

I would go to the hospital every evening in time for the evening meal, carrying my school lunch with me. Up in the lift, turn the corner, into his room – first on the left.

A face lighting up ... gold gleaming in a creek bed ...

Messages from home would be conveyed, newspapers read, tidying up attended to – then the sound of a trolley rumbling down the corridor. Hurry out! Hurry! Patients had to be quick – orders placed, food delivered to the beds all in the blink of an eyelid.

It became my mission to slow these proceedings just long enough to be able to report back to let *him* make the choice. Not unreasonable in the circumstances, I would have thought. Not according to the trolley staff though, whose prime function seemed to be to hold the line against infection. Their trolley was the barrier – I the most likely carrier. I would be waved back, glared at and muttered about. To a man and woman, their resolve to maintain those stainless-steel dishes in a state of pristine sterility never wavered, which meant, of course, that I was never supposed to look at them. I was reduced to making tiny lunges foodwards whenever the trolley staff were momentarily distracted – which was not often – but I did manage to get the odd fleeting glimpse at what was on offer.

What was on offer was pretty good. Chicken or meat cooked to as near perfection as bulk cooking will allow, a variety of vegetables, which might even include braised fennel on good nights, and a dessert course of baked apple or pear. All the vegetables and fruit were fresh – we would see them arriving at the hospital in great cartloads.

By the time Eric had finished eating, the hygiene patrol would have long departed. Sometimes the apple would be set aside for later, and I always lived in hope that the used plate, knife and fork would be cleared away by the nursing staff. A seldom-to-be-realised hope. I would scrape and clean in the hand basin – so efficiently, indeed, that one day I blocked the drain. It took days to fix, I stoutly maintaining ignorance of the cause to the end.

In the first few days, I managed to squirrel many essentials into our room – plates, knives, spoons, glasses. It took awhile, but I gradually built up a little stock, and hid it. I would raid linen trolleys – never successfully enough to find sheets for my own bed, which remained unchanged for our entire stay. Eric's bed linen had to be changed by the staff, more often than they wanted to, probably. All our difficulties, of course, were exacerbated by my inability to speak the language, and it was only when a French speaker was in attendance that real progress was made. Perhaps spreading some money around could have ushered in a few improvements. Should not this information be top of the list for consular staff to pass on, I asked myself? Flash the money! And yet, I am not so sure. I never saw any evidence of *particular* efforts being made by the staff on behalf of any patient. I am inclined to think that in this over-stretched public hospital everyone was in the same boat. No favours, anywhere.

When Eric was finally settled for the night, hair brushed, face washed, teeth cleaned, I would go down to the bar and buy a plastic cup of coffee, and then lie on my bed and open the school lunch – prosciutto, olives, bread. If I had managed to get an English newspaper I would read that to us both, and finally, unable to delay it any longer, reach the moment I had been putting off since arrival: Getting Myself Ready For Bed. For the first few nights I had brought night attire, but that swiftly degenerated to strip down to undies and wrap on an old dalmatian-spotted black and white gown. Then, reluctantly, into the bathroom, always making sure to carefully lock the sharer's door – or risk interruption. As well as stockings and other odd articles of elderly attire, I frequently shared the room with a container of her urine, which lingered for an interminable time. Presumably it was required for analysis, but what were they doing? Waiting for it to grow something? In my ensuite! My first action on entering was always to fling open the tiny window and gulp in fresh air. One night, inevitably, a sudden breeze blew the toilet roll into the bowl. A lovely moment. On another occasion the seat broke and seat and I crashed to the floor with a resounding clatter and a stream of invective. There was no response – and it was days before the seat was mended.

The very worst of tortures was when the birdlike

creature who shared the ensuite forgot to unlock *our* door when she had finished. I was always in extremis at such times, having waited far too long. So, ring for a nurse, explain the situation with the help of mime, and exercise maximum control while the nurse went round and at last unlocked the door. At times, I was desperate enough to contemplate creeping into the birdlike creature's room to open the door myself. The thought of being escorted off the premises as an intruder inhibited me.

Finally, he and I would say good night.

There were nights I would wake and realize he was awake, too. He never disturbed me, and I would feel ashamed at the thought of his being awake for goodness knew how long. I would try to soothe him to sleep. Often I would sing to him. Once my mind rocketed back to *The Ancient Mariner*, not thought of since school –

> O sleep! it is a gentle thing,
> Beloved from pole to pole!
> To Mary Queen the praise be given!

> She sent the gentle sleep from Heaven,
> That slid into my soul.

Over and over. I even set it to music. There I would be, trying everything to get him off to sleep. Stroking, soothing ...

I was singing to my baby again, but unlike my baby he would not complain if I grew weary. I did not grow weary. I would have sung all night.

With the first hint of a new day slipping into our room I would be up and at the basin. A splashing on of water, cleaning of teeth, dragging on of clothes, straightening of the bed, and the day was upon us. Down to the bar – it was always crowded at that hour with staff changing over. It became a jolly café at a railway station. I would stock up on yogurt and water from the fridge, order espresso from one counter, pay around at the other – I soon learned the system. Sometimes I would go into the unkempt garden and walk around the cloisters, sipping the hot coffee. At that hour of the day it was tranquil and beautiful. I could be in a country garden. The bells ringing, birds darting, swooping, alighting – seemingly unmindful of the cats dotted about. Those moments of isolation touched bliss ... and like the dark moments of Venice, they, too, stay with me.

Back to our room to my man, not my baby, just in time for breakfast. No choice to be made here, just rolls and terrible coffee. I would spoon the yogurt into him and the apple or pear, stay for awhile, and then say good-bye, promising to be back very quickly. The children would be there, too, I would remind him. The partings were always hard.

Next to the hospital is the church of San Giovanni e Paolo. After leaving through the great arched hospital doors, always, if I am honest, with a sense of release, I would go into the church and sit for awhile. The interior of this church is very gloomy, vast, but sometimes when the light filters through it becomes a fine theatrical space. Never quite enough light, though, if sitting, to make out Titian's *St Peter the Martyr,* which can only be seen properly, they tell me, if you have enough coins to switch on the floodlights. Enough coins and enough energy ...

I would walk back to the apartment, where three would be in various stages of rising and dressing.

Breakfast over – with the perfect toast – and then the glorious moment of standing under a shower and washing away the hospital and some of the weariness. Strains were beginning to show among the three, who were bumping into one another too much for comfort. In a few days, Jonathan would pack his swag and find a female-free zone in a charming small hotel nearer the hospital. This gave him not only a female-free living space inside, but the added joy of a tourist-free space outside. We then all got together only at the hospital or over lunch – a much better arrangement, and the apartment began to grow a little.

Easter was almost upon us.

Eric and I had specially arranged our Venetian journey to coincide with Easter. The great Christian festival and pageant was to be our goal, we decided, if we could not be in Venice for Carnevale. Easter and Carnevale – those great Venetian book ends either side of Lent. We might have had a sneaking preference for Venice at Carnevale, but Easter, we consoled ourselves, would uplift and inspire, and the music would be sublime. Much safer, too. During Carnevale we just may have lost ourselves.

Our other great Easter had been in Paris in the eighties, when a severe dose of food poisoning, due to eating at Paris's most famous restaurant, caused flights to be cancelled. We had met Kirrily in Europe and gone to Paris together to see our print dealer. Dinner was to be the treat before going our separate ways. Instead, dinner delayed us long enough for Easter Day to be celebrated in Notre Dame – where the crashing, rolling thunder of the mighty organ and the slightly panicky scramble by all in the congregation to receive the host can cause the faint-hearted to swoon. I hid behind a pillar – crowds, as ever, my phobia. The service over, we bought a CD to revisit the sound and finally emerged into the sunshine, unable to speak.

Easter in Venice, we knew, would equal this other high point in our spiritual lives.

Anna and Jane woke early to the sound of the bells. They went to San Marco before the crowds, their only companions a group of nuns singing their joy. They lit candles, as they always did now, and had returned to the apartment by the time I arrived. We had decided to eat at the apartment – Jonathan cooking – so before going back to the hospital the girls and I went to the Rialto and found the pasta shop, already crowded with Venetians who knew precisely what they wanted from the bewildering array of shapes and sizes and colours. We felt like novices, but finally settled on shape, and colour, and went to another shop for chocolates, somewhere else for bread. Jonathan was searching out the ingredients for his sauce and collecting the wine. On our way back, via San Marco, I slipped into the side chapel and sat gazing at my Madonna with her ancient, wise infant. I was, as ever, utterly focused, my prayer, through her, modest – Just let us get him out of Venice. Then I lit *my* candle.

We set off, all four, to the hospital, collecting an armful of iris on the way, great iris blue stems. We went into his room bringing the gift of our love.

And there was Eric, lying on a bed, festooned with drips, paralysed down one side, able to communicate only with difficulty. There was Eric, landed slap bang into the middle of an Easter neither of us in our wildest nightmares could have imagined.

Easter, nonetheless . . .

'Can you just hear those bells, Dad?' from Anna.

'That's what I've been trying to say to you for days! They're driving me crazy!' And he picked up the high-tech hearing aid, put it in his ear, and instructed Anna in the tricky business of adjusting the volume.

A huge smile. He had just had another Easter present.

We left him, finally, after supervising his lunch, putting the iris in the basin so he would see them; said we would be back soon.

There was a table against the wall in the apartment. As always, it was covered with clothes, books. We cleared it and put it in the centre of the room, found a tablecloth, and napkins, and turned it into something festive while Jonathan cooked. The meal was delicious,

I remember, and the wine. What did we talk about? I think Jonathan and I might have pointed the girls in the direction of the paintings, sculptures, churches they should see in spare moments. The consul, Charles Farrugia, rang to say he would be visiting Eric the next day, and we invited him back to the flat for coffee. We had spoken to Sydney earlier, as it was Easter – though everyone avoided mentioning the fact.

Lunch over, we walked back through the crowds to the hospital and told Eric that Charles would be visiting tomorrow, which delighted him. We put the iris in a container and placed it on the window sill. There was a vase on the sill of the room on the other side of the garden – not iris, but neatly symmetrical. Pleasing. We talked about what it would be like when we got him home, how plans were progressing. We talked about the spring weather, which changed every time we came out now. We brought him many, many messages. We tried to catch some of the Primario's spirit –

'I am always optimistic.'

I think we succeeded – at least in fooling him …

I am walking across the second-last bridge. My feelings are close to despair. There will be no escape from Venice. I know that now. The children cannot put their lives on hold forever. I do not know what will happen. I do not know how I will manage.

Approaching are two young people. They recognize me, so that means they are Australian. They are full of excitement and joy and abundant life. That is what I notice, their abundant life. I want to scrape some off and spread it all over me. And then, seduced by their intelligence – their bright, gleaming intelligence – I find I am telling them my story.

I am here in Venice with my critically ill husband, I tell them. I am living in an apartment at the moment, but I shall have to leave shortly. What on earth I shall be doing then I have not the faintest idea. In a flash, bubbling out of them is a description of their quite perfect accommodation. They have rooms in a faded palazzo owned by an eccentric Russian who had been an intimate of Peggy Guggenheim. Every morning, they breakfast with her, and she tells them stories of life in Venice when Venice was Venice, not the hotch-potch of tourism that it is now. They listen to her tales open mouthed and are in serious danger of not ever seeing any sort of Venice because this woman of some mystery – she changes her name occasionally, depending on the mood – has them in thrall. The place is perfect, they assure me, and they pass over her address and say good-bye, fascinated all over again by an encounter with me on the second-last bridge. I think in Venice they have stacked up much ammunition for dinner parties back home.

As I leave them, my spirits have lifted and I enter the world of Peggy Guggenheim's intimate, where breakfasts are shared and I travel to the hospital with lots of stories for Eric, and where my daily pacings through this city of masks will begin to include, doubtless, visits to a bar. There will be an increasing interest in absinthe. I will become part of the city, slightly mysterious – pointed out to tourists.

Jane is walking across the campo outside the hospital, having just visited her father. Her head is bowed, she is alone in the world, an expatriate, not a traveller. Lost in thought. On the opposite side of the campo, on his way to work, the Primario sees her. He swerves and strides across, takes her in his arms, hugs her for a moment or two, and then disappears without a word through the great arched doorway.

We are, all four, looking for a restaurant for lunch. It has been a perfect Venetian spring day, when a sudden storm blows up and we are being pelted with hail. We race with the crowds. Every restaurant fills in an instant, but we finally squeeze into one, drenched, and watch in amazement and with a sense of fun as the hail bounces over paving stones and quickly empties the campos. In an hour, the sun is out again, but it will be raining that night on the way to the hospital. The first item to pack for Venice must always be an umbrella . . .

On the way back from San Marco I go into a café and stand at the counter for an espresso. Eric and I had gone there in the mornings of that first week, after early walks. They serve breakfasts and lunches, but standing at the counter ordering the espresso is the Venetian way. This day, two policemen come in. They have been tramping the beat. They don't need to order. Two espressos and two glasses of water are placed on the high counter. They sip their coffee. They drink the water, solemnly conversing. They replace their tiny cups on the counter and stroll out into the calle. No money has been exchanged. I see them many times after this. They are very suave.

I am sitting at the desk in the apartment, looking out the window. I watch the man in his shop on the left of the canal. A small shop given over to the making of chairs. He manipulates the cane, polishes the wood, bends and shapes. They are simple chairs, and when he finishes one he hangs it outside his shop above the pavement. He has two assistants who work in shifts. The assistant will bring a cart along, load up the chairs and push the cart around the corner. He vanishes in seconds. Sometimes, chairs are carried to a mooring post and loaded onto a boat. So much work, so much effort to get the chairs to their destination, which, when reached, will surely involve climbing up four flights. I watch him shut up his shop in the middle of the day. Fine weather, fair weather, foul weather. Old ladies with their small dogs in tow pass his shop. Sometimes, one will stop at the door to the right of his. She uses her key, enters, closes the door behind her. I know she, too, will then be labouring up three or four flights, for she would not be living at canal level like uninformed travellers. How tough these old Venetian women are. The apartment at the top of that building has window boxes, where, among the burgeoning seedlings, tiny windmills whirr. It is hoped these enchanting little toys will discourage the pigeons.

I yearn to see Venice in winter. I shall never go to Venice again . . .

In another life, Eric and I are walking around the Doge's Palace. Eric has taken photographs; we look at everything. We are tourists. Many people about, but not crushingly so. There is a group of young boys being taken around by their teacher. He is a very ordinary-looking man – middle-aged, average, nothing to distinguish him from the many other teachers we have seen leading groups of all ages through Venice and around the treasures. Except . . .

his boys are speeding through every corner, coming to abrupt halts, looking, really looking, at everything they see, constantly flying back to him with individual questions, individual comments. Their faces are alight, their energy boundless. Sometimes they all gather around him and he talks at length. They drink in everything he tells them, dash off again, sometimes alone, sometimes in pairs, sometimes staying in a group. Their chief delight is to share with him. His chief delight is to teach. They absorb, they grow, they open out – they are bursting out of their buds. We watch it happening and something rubs off – a light dusting of pollen perhaps. These boys do not have to be disciplined. Their flight around the Palace offends none. Wherever they alight they give pleasure. I think to myself that to be a great teacher is the most rewarding job in the world. A direct, unwavering, reliable track …

There is a shop we four sometimes pass on our way to a restaurant after the morning hospital visit. It is on the corner of a campo and sells masks, scraps of costume, posters, religious or bizarre – sometimes both. Outside the shop stand dummies draped in silks and frills, some with chiffon hemlines stiffened into extravagant shapes. The attire is undoubtedly female, the dummies indisputably male. They wear strange embroidered skullcaps with nobs on the top. Most have shoulder-length white hair. Their faces are old, stern and chilling. High white stilt heels are on their feet. One is bare chested with a reproduction of his goatee-bearded face tattooed onto the chest, like a bleeding heart. Another, with short hair and a hip-length, beautifully coloured and patterned silk jacket, has a representation of the Virgin on his chest. Their arms are akimbo, their stance and mien aggressive. Seen together, or singly, the impression is nightmarish. They fit into our lives quite comfortably at the moment.

On Easter Monday, Charles Farrugia, the consul, interrupts his holiday and visits Eric. Later, he and his wife come to the apartment for coffee. It is a most pleasant meeting, and he thinks Eric's spirits are fine. We talk of many things – life back in Sydney, theatre and opera, their life in Rome, their responsibilities, and we are assured of all help as the days – weeks? – progress. Their visit has brought a welcome breath of normalcy to our lives. We will have every assistance from the Consulate while we are here and when, hopefully, the time arrives for our departure. We are not alone, Charles assures us. Coffee over, we bid them good-bye. They depart. We wave. They disappear around the corner of Corte Gregolini, mobile at the ready, as they prepare to resume their holiday. We have had a social occasion! It feels quite strange – but very comforting. We are *not* alone in Italy. Pity it is Venice, though. These calamities should only happen in Rome.

Eric has now been in hospital for nearly two weeks. We spend as much time as is needed in the Primario's office, and he advises that Eric is getting a little stronger and perhaps in a week we can begin to look at the possibility of his return to Sydney. We dare not take this as a certainty, but, at last, there is a little hope. When he travels it will be a medical evacuation, and the ramifications of this will be explained to us nearer the time. Insurance, which of course we have, will cover the extremely expensive procedure. We all have a goal now – a goal Eric is determined to reach.

I continue to marvel at his sanguine acceptance of what is a terrible predicament. Very little causes him to lose patience, let alone good humour. He is extraordinary.

With, it must be confessed, just the one exception. We have one area of almighty conflict – his highly expensive, high-tech, state-of-the-art, beautifully constructed, skilfully able to be concealed in the ear hearing aid, which is developing, and will continue to develop, into a dangerous bone of contention between us. Cursed with an absence of manual dexterity of any kind, the minute adjustments called for, the delicate able-to-pick-a-lock digital manoeuvrings required to make the fucking thing work are beyond me. I am happy to confess my inadequacies, ready to resign my position at any time, but of course that is no help – there being no one else standing in line waiting for the privilege, if I happen to be visiting him alone.

Eric, on these occasions, is impossible. With his somewhat limited vocabulary, he gets as close to browbeating me as has ever occurred in our entire marriage. He gets close simply because he is so ill.

My patience is heroic. Calmly, I endeavour to work my way through the ramifications of the minute adjustments required. Returned to him, inserted, there is an outraged 'No! It's no good!' from him. I clean it, or try to, say prayers over it, wave the singed tail feathers of roosters above it, tell him to wait for the children ... it might work for a tiny period, then the whole business starts up again. As his hearing seems to have improved remarkably since the stroke, I feel he is being extremely unreasonable. Things seem to proceed very happily with the device sitting there on his bedside table.

The greatest trauma of all is occasioned by its disappearance in the bed. Trying to retrieve a tiny object in these circumstances is not to be recommended – particularly if the device has disappeared seconds before a sudden onrush of enthusiasm has prompted the nursing staff to change the bedding.

This aside, my beloved is flawless. Unbeatable. Sensational. Olympian.

APRIL 14: It is quiet at the hospital. Eric has settled down for the night. We are, as always, disturbed briefly throughout the night as nurses make their rounds, checking to see that patients are safe – and alive, presumably. Torches shine in faces. Doors close. Sometimes a bag that drips life in needs to be changed; sometimes vital monitoring takes place. I am in a deep sleep, dreamless, unconscious. Nothing will wake me. But of course it does. It is the sickening sound of a crash, and I am up in a flash, ringing for help even before switching on my light because I know it is serious. I cannot see him in his bed. I think I must be going mad ... I cannot see him because he is on the floor on the other side. Stands carrying drips are overturned and in the slow motion of my reaching him I do not even know if he will be alive when I get to him, or why he is on the floor. He is on the floor because he has fallen out of bed. Almost as I reach him the door flies open and in a second his room is full of nurses and someone is summoning night duty doctors and they arrive very, very quickly. He *is* alive and I am ordered out, still struggling into the dalmatian gown, and his slippers, which I have worn since I came here as they are comfortable and made of fine, soft leather – and

I do not own any. The door is closed firmly behind me and I pace and pace, up and down the corridor, sometimes going into the waiting room at the end where a few sleepy nearest and dearest wait out the night. I feel sick and I am terribly, terribly apprehensive and I cannot believe any of it. After an eternity, the door opens, the captains depart and a young nurse smiles and tells me he is all right and I may return. He had fallen straight onto his nose, it seems, which must have been – and still is, doubtless – extremely painful. But he smiles at me, and I cannot believe how patient this patient is. I take the hand that is free of leads, but which is now a little more difficult to get at, because the sides of the bed have been put on. They have made sure, now, that he will not fall out again.

The next day we learn that his nose is fractured. Worse, that it must be operated upon before he can fly. This is to be done at the earliest possible opportunity. A minor operation and there should be no problems. I think there is a vast sense of relief all around Internal Medicine. Greater damage from the fall – a not unlikely possibility – would have wiped out all chance of evacuation. All staff at San Giovanni e Paolo, from the Primario down, are desperately working to bring us a happy ending.

It is around about this time that arrangements are being entered into with the insurers. I should say we are *endeavouring* to enter into arrangements. From the outset, we are met with obstruction, rudeness, and a refusal on the part of the only contact available, the managing director of the organization, to accept the seriousness of Eric's situation. This person is also the only one to answer the organization's emergency number, and his response, if unfortunately awakened by a phone call from us when we are in extremis, is to insist that our case is not an emergency at all. Why are we waking him? So begins a war of attrition, slowly at first, because no one really believes that obligations will – or can – be avoided, but more and more heatedly as the days pass, and we begin to catch a glimpse of a certainty that until then had seemed too fragile to pin hopes on. Namely, that we *will* be embarking on a medical evacuation.

APRIL 16: This is the day they operate on Eric's nose. When he returns from the operating theatre, his nose is packed with dressing, and plaster stretches across his face. He lies quietly. We do not speak.

Eric has had a stroke, he suffers from a yet unexplained blood disorder, which has his life balanced on a knife edge, and his nose has been broken. He also has a spot on his lung – though, hopefully, this is a diminishing problem with the help of antibiotics. I think he has had more than enough, but find I am crossing my fingers, in the Venetian way, to persuade the fates to leave him alone for awhile.

APRIL 19: Jonathan is undertaking a brief day trip to Florence to see an old friend who runs a charter helicopter organization there. It is a very Venetian spring day, though perhaps the weather vane these past few days is swinging more towards rain ... and more rain. The bursts of bright sunlight are lessening, though for us weather sinks in importance in the overall scheme of things. I remember lunch that day in a very small restaurant, sitting outside, but being forced to keep an eye on the sky so the dash to safety would just beat the drenching. We are in a tiny, paved area, a branch of a tree softening the wall at the side. Leaves not out yet but one feels their imminence. We are in a state of torpor. The time has approached for my daughters to leave us. This sits heavily. They have found the private garden alongside San Marco and tell me I must see it. It is the most beautiful garden in Venice, they insist. I say yes I must, knowing I will not.

I have found some wonderful blood oranges today. These give Eric the greatest of pleasure. He will love these ones. I leave the girls, who will go to the hospital a little later, and stride in with my prize. Carefully, I peel an orange and sit beside the bed, popping segment after segment into his mouth. These are the best oranges in the world; the juice drips down my arms as I tear the segments. I could wish that the juice were another colour. There has been enough blood about us. When I first found the oranges, the bag under his bed matched them more nearly. He is improving. As I feed him he emits tiny sounds of appreciation and we discuss their excellence. His delight is infectious and I steal the occasional bite. It is sweet – so sweet! These are the times we need nothing else. We are happy, Eric and I. The golden orange with its bloody centre creates its own magic. We are wrapped in it, soothed by it and alone in the world.

Fifteen months later I am watching an innocent cooking programme on television. The cook, Stefano Di Pieri, is bicycling through the Riverina and he is going to visit a friend. It is the most idyllic of scenes, reminiscent of Tuscany. A meandering dirt road turns around a bend, revealing a splendid orchard of orange trees, and long before the cook cuts into the fruit I know they will be blood oranges and I am engulfed in such a deep and animal grief that had it been witnessed or heard, those not yet experienced in these matters would have been at pains to comprehend the spectacle. Minutes later, the tempest has vanished as erratically as it appeared. These are the ways of grief.

Jonathan has collected his compact rent-a-Fiat. He drives south, is reunited with his friend, Alain, in Florence and they head for the village of San Gimignano for lunch. On a crest in the road, two motor cyclists race past them and are met head on by a Range Rover. A double fatality, which I do not hear about for quite some time, though I remember when I asked him how his day was he remarked cryptically, 'Life's a knife edge!'

APRIL 20: We have a meeting with the Primario. He had indicated the possibility at the end of last week, but now confirms, that we should aim for a medical evacuation of Eric on Friday of this week – April 24. Eric has progressed to the stage where, barring the blood becoming uncontrollable again, he should be in a fit enough state to manage the journey. But there should be no delay. We are to confirm this date with the travel insurers in Australia and arrangements will be put in hand to book a doctor and nurse, much of whose life, seemingly, is spent travelling the world on these hazardous journeys. The Consulate will be notified and all the ramifications that accompany such an operation will be set in motion. As ever, our Primario is supremely confident that all will proceed according to plan. The adrenalin begins to hit a new high.

Meanwhile, the rain has set in in Venice. Intermittent for days, it showed its true calibre round about the time of Eric's operation. Walking along narrow calles is difficult. It has become a business of umbrella jousting with umbrella, a flattening of bodies against walls, and water seemingly everywhere, not just in canals. At breakfast that morning I watch as the canal edges up over the steps near the chairmaker's shop and gives every indication of beginning to lap onto the paving in front. I walk out into the entrance hall of our building and see that the water is well and truly under the canal doors and over the steps, and I decide not to speculate on how long, if things do not improve, it would take to enter our apartment and invade our belongings. All this and aqua alta, too! Don't think! Don't think! We have been using two of Nicole's umbrellas ever since our three children arrived in Venice. 'You don't need to buy umbrellas, Mrs Phillips. Take these for the time being.' Yes, Nicole. Anna and Jane are leaving tomorrow, so they have arranged to say good-bye and hand over the umbrellas (Jonathan had bought an extremely swish Italian one for himself very early in the piece, which went beautifully with his torn Armani jeans).

Nicole arrives. We have seen her many times over the past two weeks, but more and more briefly and always with discretion, because she knows that my great need for her diminished with their arrival. She has been on call twenty-four hours a day, if necessary. So the farewells are emotional, like all farewells that end something special. And this has been *so* special for all of us, not least Nicole, who has been deeply affected by Eric's trouble. She has maintained her visits to him, and in the process of encouragement and service and the brightening up of his day has entered his pantheon of special women – a select group.

Anna and Jane and Nicole make their farewells and I take advantage of the moment for a photo opportunity out in the corte in front of the fountain. We leave her and head for the hospital – a suitable break in the weather making it possible without extra umbrellas.

Another emotional time looms, much deeper this one. The girls farewell Eric, trying to keep their tears in check – 'Just remember! We'll see you on *Sunday!*' 'I'll *be* there!' he says to them, raising his clenched left fist. They leave him and arrive at the lift just as I step out. They are both in floods of tears by now, much to the consternation of the Primario, who has been holding a corridor meeting with colleagues –

'What is this? What is this?' he says. 'Surely my patient hasn't died! That can be the only reason for such tears!' They smile at last and assure him that his patient continues well. But he then says, 'Remember! The spot on his lung is unchanged.' I do not hear him say this.

APRIL 21: Anna and Jane leave with an extra bag – Eric's – full of his clothes and any book I can lay my hands on. We do not even contemplate excess. A chapter ends. I feel desolate but am comforted by the thought that barring – I resist saying accidents – but barring any setback we will be together again very shortly. Jonathan escorts them to the airport. They will spend a night at a hotel in Rome (later reported as drab and depressing in the extreme) and then board the flight for Sydney. I am faced with a major problem as the apartment needs to be vacated on Thursday and we are scheduled to leave on Friday morning. This is very unfortunate timing, but already we have been able to stay much longer than originally intended. I begin the final pack, dreading the prospect of us getting my bag plus extras over to Jonathan's hotel, where the kind owners have agreed to put us up for one night in the bridal suite – which, due to an influx of tourists, is the only space available. I cannot wait for this Oedipal development. Jonathan is swift to advise that the bridal bed transforms into twins in a flash.

The insurer in Sydney seems to have arrived at a stage of mulish unhelpfulness. The agencies in London and Zurich, who are handling arrangements for him in the northern hemisphere, are becoming anxious as no money has as yet been transferred. Bookings have been made with Alitalia, but the seats cannot be held indefinitely. A medical evacuation that includes doctor and nurse requires an allocation of nine seats, plus two for Jonathan and me. We are well aware that Friday is the one window of opportunity.

Now begins an agonizing process of pushing Sydney, persuading Alitalia to hold the seats, and keeping the doctor and nurse on standby while everything is sorted out. Rita at the Consulate has become vital. She is in constant communication with all parties, including the Primario and Dr Busetto. And she is also in communication with Jonathan. Her voice, which I have come to know very well ('Do not worry, Mrs Phillips. You must not worry.'), is the best voice in the world. What I do not know during this week is that one of her main refrains to Jonathan is, 'Don't tell your mother, Jonathan! Don't tell your mother!', as matters descend further and further into the abyss. On this Tuesday night, Jonathan returns to our apartment, takes his father's half bottle of vodka out of the fridge, sits down and phones the world. This is the night that Dr Busetto is on the phone, too, as medical information is required in Zurich and London. What no one knows is that Jonathan and I will get Eric out of Venice on Friday *no matter what.* Jonathan is arranging for enough money to be made available to enable us to front up with two bits of plastic – his and mine – which will allow us to set off. All of us! We will think about the debt later. We do not intend to let that window be slammed shut on us.

By the time the night is over, the vodka bottle is empty.

APRIL 22: I stay at the hospital longer in the morning. Breakfast at the apartment holds few joys. It has occurred to me that I have no idea of Jonathan's address. If he returned to his hotel in the early hours of the morning, which is more than likely, I shall have to wait till we meet up at the hospital before I can be sure he has not been mugged. If he has been, no one can bring us together again for quite awhile! I dismiss the thought, too unpleasant. Why do I never worry about him when I am not with him? Three years in Nigeria and I did not have a moment's unease – apart from the time he had typhoid and malaria in tandem. But the political turmoil caused me never a tremor.

Dr Busetto has come in to check reports. The packing has been removed from Eric's nose. She is engrossed but I interrupt her concentration. 'Coraggioso,' I say, looking at him. She pauses for a moment, giving me her cool gaze, and then, 'The whole family – coraggioso.' We look at one another for a few seconds until she returns to familiar territory among the reports.

I bid Eric good-bye. He is aware a momentous day is approaching and seems entirely focused on conserving his energy and willing himself fitter. I abandon the idea of breakfast at the apartment and go into the bar at the end of our calle. It is apparently the very best in Venice and we only made that discovery a week ago! Never mind. The coffee is blissful, as is the croissant – which I never eat in Sydney. I stand with commuters and the inevitable dog or two, mostly small at this end of town. *Two* coffees.

More sorting out to do. I cannot get any money – the bloody card will not work. Never mind. At least order prevails in the apartment – most of the packing done. The absent owner of the flat will be greatly relieved to be finally shot of us, I imagine, though in our few brief phone conversations she has been sympathetic and generous. She herself has been delayed in

Rome because her husband – a government senator – had been rushed off to hospital about the same time as Eric, with pneumonia. What *is* it about this place?

Our doctor in Sydney, Barbara Jenner, has organized for an ambulance to meet our flight. Her husband will be in charge at Emergency in the Adventist Hospital in Wahroonga, which is Eric's destination, so it is all in the family and there will be a familiar face for Eric. A neurologist, a haematologist, and a lung specialist will be waiting, if not all there on the Sunday, certainly by the Monday.

Crossed fingers! Crossed fingers!

When I return to the hospital, Jonathan, to my great relief, is there, after an uneventful if solitary return to his dwelling in the small hours. There is still no resolution of the insurance problem. Rita is never off the phone. If she speaks to me it is always, 'Do not worry, Mrs Phillips!' If she speaks to Jonathan, it is, 'Don't tell your mother, Jonathan!' We have no guarantees, and the agents in the northern hemisphere, while absolutely helpful and courteous, are, understandably, nervous about finalising everything before they see the colour of the Sydney money. Rita, in some mysterious way known only to her, is managing to convince Alitalia that there is nothing whatever to worry about.

Tonight will be my last night sleeping at the hospital. I have explained to Eric that there is too much to organize, and getting the luggage to the hospital on Friday morning will require much effort and wit.

I kiss him and settle for my last night at San Giovanni e Paolo, surprised that I do so with a complete lack of emotion.

APRIL 23: It is the middle of the afternoon on this Thursday. Jonathan and I have taken my bag plus extras to his hotel – up and over the bridges. No porter in evidence, of course, and my right foot starting to nag ominously. I ignore it. Where he has been staying is peaceful after the environs of Corte Gregolini. The narrowest of passageways connecting through a maze of confusingly identical buildings, most of them dwellings. He takes me into a wonderful bespoke printery, Il Papiro, where at least one of the printing presses dates back centuries. It is owned by a charming man, who prints cards and writing paper for clients all over the world. He asks me why on earth I have been staying near San Marco! This is the *real* Venice he assures me – and of course he is right. I buy some cards, lose myself for ten minutes or so in the sort of tranquillity I had forgotten about. Earlier, we had entered a doorway set in a grey wall, identical to its neighbour (How do roistering travellers find their own burrow late at night?), which is Jonathan's hotel. The doorway opens into a tiny garden with a fountain in a niche at one end, bulbs in bloom, a cherry tree, a pile of strawberries scattered on one of the tables. I look round for easel and painter – everything quiet, quiet, including the voices of the welcoming hosts who are, of course, aware of our situation.

That morning, we had been to the bank and prized some money out of them; returned to the apartment and settled accounts with Nicole. I gave her a pair of earrings intended for Gully in Majorca. This good-bye was not easy, but I said I would be thinking of her and her Italian husband in the Seychelles. There was no point in trying to articulate what her presence had meant to me in those early horrifying days ... no need to ... any words meaningless ... we both knew, anyway. Ciao, Nicole.

We have the money for the journey! Finally, it has come down to the insurer proffering his Diners Club number. The agents here give the word to proceed.

Extraordinary! It is extraordinary, wonderful, hair-raising, reckless, it is five minutes to midnight – but it is ...

At the hospital, all is being made ready. Jonathan has the necessary paperwork advising that Eric is indeed fit enough to get on the plane, as long as he has doctor and nurse in attendance. Forget these papers and forget getting out of Venice. There are reports, x-rays and scans to accompany him. The doctor and nurse are with Eric at the moment and we meet them in the Primario's office. They are remarkably and comfortingly ordinary. Eric's doctor is Michael Pagliero. He is from Dover – where, it seems, he is quite an exponent of organ playing. His nurse is from Hull. The only thing to lift her out of the English matter-of-factness of Hull, perhaps, is her surname, which is unmistakably Arabic and which will present an unforeseen difficulty further down the track. Her first name is Sylvia. These two manage to give the impression that a medical evacuation is as simple as a trip to the supermarket, which, to them, I daresay it is. We arrange to meet at eight o'clock in the morning, ready to leave. Jonathan and Sylvia will travel together by taxi, taking the luggage with them; Michael and I will follow with Eric. Already my stomach is a swarm of butterflies! Before we leave, we give the Primario the beautiful wooden book ends originally intended for Tim in Majorca. He is touched and delighted.

Eric is quiet and fully prepared. And completely aware of the enormity of the journey ahead. We can see him conserving, conserving ... He does not particularly want to talk. We are all a little solemn. Jonathan and I leave.

We look for somewhere to eat, and finally it is a bar that serves meals. It is crowded and we have to stand at the bar for some time, sipping. Noise, but cheerful, happy noise, and the plates of steaming food look scrumptious. I could not care less, but food seems essential. At last we are squeezed into a corner somewhere, plates arrive, are dealt with, and whether it was good or bad I cannot say. We leave the crowd to their jollity and walk slowly back to Jonathan's hotel, are admitted to the secret garden and climb the winding steps to the bridal suite. The bed is now two, but cheek by jowl, for this bridal suite is minuscule. We cannot move about at the same time, our luggage having robbed the room of what space it had. All must be in perfect order for the morning, clothes on the ends of the beds, everything at the ready for an early and swift departure. What I mean is the *slowest* because, again, all luggage has to be transported, except for my cabin bag, by my poor son. And so to bed.

APRIL 24: We creep out just after six o'clock, I carrying my cabin bag. Jonathan is striding ahead, even with two suitcases, and I have to keep telling him to slow down, because if he disappears *I* will never be seen again. His humour is not the sunniest. There is not a soul to be seen as we head towards the hospital – then, as I glance to my left, a hundred metres away, Nicole has materialised. I cannot believe my eyes. Why is she here? This is not where she lives.

It is a snapshot. The composition is perfect. I hear 'Good luck, Mrs Phillips. Good luck!' And the snapshot vanishes. Like the Cheshire Cat. How extraordinary! But then – why not? Only to be expected ...

The hospital. Finally. We try to persuade two members of staff in Emergency to mind our bags for a short time. They are monumentally uninterested, but we leave the bags anyway. Jonathan makes one more trip to the bridal suite; I make for the bar and stock up on yogurt and one coffee for me, and take the lift for the last time to Internal Medicine. There is much activity, as they are getting Eric ready. I am leaning against the corridor wall, holding the yogurts. My cabin bag is alongside. It is a beautiful spring day, beautiful enough for umbrellas to be packed. A nurse calls me and I go in. They have lifted Eric into a wheelchair and she asks me to hold him. I greet him; he is very quiet. My hand is on his shoulder, and then he begins to slump in the chair and next my arms are around him trying desperately to hold him in the chair and at the same time shouting for help. Two nurses run in and I yell at them to get him back on the bed, and Dr Busetto flies in and I know she is in the mightiest panic as she says over and over again, 'Mr Phillips! Mr Phillips! You must be well! You have to leave here!' And *I* know they have wrecked it and we are not going to get out! At the eleventh hour we are not going to get out of this hospital! We are in Venice forever! I am striding the corridor shouting 'Stupido! Stupido!' The bird-like creature is at her door. *All* doors are opening. It is pandemonium in Eric's room. And I think to myself, 'You've blown it, all of you! You've wrecked us! One senseless action of putting him in a chair, and you've done us ... Oh, God! Oh, God!' I am Hecuba, I am Clytemnestra ... I am finished ...

It is peaceful in his room. Dr Michael Pagliero arrives. They have summoned him. If he decides Eric's blood pressure has regained an acceptable level he will agree to take him. Not otherwise. I am slumped on the wall and have no hope whatsoever.

Michael emerges. We will go. We must be accompanied by blood and plasma, but we will go – of course. He seems perfectly calm. Everything is calm. Quiet ... The storms are over. But I think Dr Busetto has aged over the last ten minutes or so. I am emptied of everything.

Then around the corner from the lift strolls our Primario.

He is not required to be here this early. He has come to farewell us.

He has stepped straight out of a Visconti film. He is in a cream suit, a coat slung around his shoulders. Debonair. He goes in to say good-bye to Eric, and they have their usual noisy and warm greeting. I can see him sitting on the bed, holding Eric's hand. Then he comes out and takes up his post on the other wall. We are all waiting ...

At last, a stretcher arrives; a sister is in charge now, supervising the careful lifting and placement of the patient.

I look over at the Primario and he winks at me and I think, I do not want to leave you. He eases himself off the wall, comes over and embraces me, kissing me on both cheeks, and after a moment I do leave. *He* knows things. There are things *I* have still to learn.

Down at water's edge, the ambulance awaits. Jonathan and Sylvia have long departed, and I watch while everything is made ready. The stretcher is lifted on board, and as it goes the sister suddenly turns and embraces me. There are tears in her eyes as she scuttles off. They may remember us at San Giovanni e Paolo for a day or two. I climb aboard, Michael and I settle as best we can and the ambulance heads off into the lagoon. The cemetery island, San Michele, looks breathtakingly beautiful in the early morning light, the bank of cypresses cutting sharply upwards. Ha! I say to myself. You didn't get him after all!

The ambulance noses gently into the wharf at the airport. Eric will be transferred to the stretcher that will be his home till he arrives at the Sydney Adventist Hospital. It seems a perilously long way off. We are not speaking much. Soon, we are in the first-aid/ambulance area of Venice airport and being greeted by a charming young doctor who is intrigued by this, possibly his first, experience of a medical evacuation. All the paperwork is in order and it now becomes a matter of waiting for the domestic flight to be ready for take-off. The first-aid area is spotless, beautifully fitted out, and I take the opportunity to give Eric some yogurt. He is complaining about missing breakfast. 'Join the club,' I say, spooning coffee yogurt into him while scoffing down my tub. He is, of course, flat on his back, the position he will be in for most of the next thirty hours or so.

I take advantage of the pristine facilities and suddenly we are moving, or rather Eric is. Sylvia, Michael and Jonathan have been about their bureaucratic affairs, the luggage has been despatched all the way to Sydney, and I am left with the airport doctor, wondering who will be getting *me* to the plane. No one seems concerned about this, and I am tiring of discussing the delights of Sydney with someone whose responsibility has now ended. I think it is more than likely the plane will take off without me, judging by the mishaps to date. However I *am* transported – by ambulance, no other vehicle being around at the time. It seems appropriate. Sylvia and Michael are already in the plane, making sure everything is proceeding. In a medical evacuation, passengers are held up until the patient is installed. We sense their impatience.

Our patient is being lifted skywards on a special forklift device that will place him adjacent to the plane door. With a strip of plaster covering his nose from one side of his face to the other and a strip over his brow, he looks more like an accident victim. I see him carried inside and am then, myself, invited to join the plane – where I am reunited with my son. We take our seats on the opposite side of the aisle to Eric's stretcher, which is placed alongside the windows. It takes up three rows, with Michael and Sylvia spreading themselves over the aisle seats. It all works, apart from the unfinished coffee yogurt emptying itself down my trouser leg. We are off!

As we circle for landing at Rome I remember that it is now my least favourite airport. Eric and his medical duo will be taken by ambulance to Rome's first-aid/ambulance area, where they will remain till it is time to board the international flight. Jonathan and I are to be met. We land; the plane stops; we say good-bye to Eric; we walk to the terminal.

At the entrance, a small crowd waits. Two faces leap out at us – Teraseta and Rita. One is carrying a mobile, so this must be Rita. We are welcomed with the utmost warmth, and are then treated to the best performance of slipping and weaving through red tape, police, security – anyone or anything that could impede our progress – that I have ever witnessed. Rita is masterful. She picks her mark, charms, flatters, cajoles, and has us waved through any possible hindrance in seconds flat. People, even the sourest, fall over themselves to be helpful.

What I do notice is that when some particularly daring manoeuvre has been accomplished, Rita returns to make a graceful speech of thanks that would have Godzilla eating out of her hand. Hers is a rare gift – and I have been with experts. The mobile is constantly, but discreetly, in use. In no time at all, we are in a consular car and being driven to my husband, who is awaiting us, supine, in a cramped corridor of the first-aid section. There, too, are Michael and Sylvia, Michael with the troubling news that the manila envelope carrying reports and leads has vanished in the scramble to disembark. Rita taps into the mobile, contacts Venice, who instigate a search of all areas of that airport. They eventually call back, but they have not found a manila envelope. This is not good, but we all smile. Rita makes one more call.

The time for departure draws near and we leave Eric, Michael and Sylvia, and are driven around Italy to the departure lounge. Rita, Teraseta and I chat of this and that, and Jonathan phones Lisa in Bondi. Then a woman wanders among the crowds holding something aloft. Rita flies off in her direction and returns with the missing envelope, rescued minutes before from the tarmac beneath our first aircraft! Mission impossible, but a pushover for Rita. We are invited to board. More farewells and I stammer inadequate thanks. From consul down, Rome has done us proud.

Eric is installed by the time we board. He is positioned in the seats just to the front of the bulkhead in Economy. His narrow stretcher wedges in cosily along the three window seats. A curtain can be pulled to give him privacy. He can be propped up into a sitting position if he feels like it, but he spends most of the journey flat on his back. Michael and Sylvia take the aisle seat near him and the paraphernalia of the medical evacuation, plus their cabin baggage, spreads out over the remaining seats. Blood and plasma are at the ready and Michael, overjoyed and mightily relieved, has been reunited with the large manila envelope. Jonathan is across the aisle from them all, and I am up front. Due to Eric's positioning it is just a short walk for me to get to him.

It is an odd situation. The social niceties elude us, and conversation, as we wait for take-off, dries up after a time. It has not taken long to exhaust the parameters of life in Dover, Hull, and previous evacuations – which would presumably have a sameness about them after a time, barring, and again I hesitate to use the word, accidents. The patient shows no inclination to contribute, but is hard to ignore, being, as he is, the centrepiece. The most intriguing information to pass among the teacups is that Michael will be performing a major thoracic operation immediately upon his return to Dover. I pray that, for his patient's sake, he continues a stranger to jet lag. Playing the organ must be the secret.

Sylvia would fit perfectly into a corner store in Hull, measuring out the biscuits and lollies while stalwartly resisting change and the encroachment of the supermarket. Instead, she flies around the world with the ill, the badly damaged, the dying. The world, I am finding, is full of the most fascinating people, and my experience of it, to date, minimal.

The captain pays a visit, satisfies himself that Eric is comfortable, and assures us of all assistance. The group occupying the seats on the other side of the bulkhead are a cheerful group of Italians who nod sympathetically in our direction. I am beginning to find the situation too difficult, pat Eric a couple of times, and retire to comparative, but quite unashamed, luxury. I sink into the seat and close my eyes ...

We are flying over Rome. I look out of the window. All the majestic landmarks stand out. We circle. I gaze and gaze ...

Without warning I am filled with a sadness such as I have never known before, and sobs thrust up from my gut – soundless, overwhelming. They run their course. I return to normal, if that is what it is called, as Jonathan moves up the aisle. He is smiling, wolf eyes gleaming, as he plonks down next to me. Someone has suggested an upgrade.

The flight between Rome and Bangkok is measured by walks up the aisle with treats for Eric, not too many of which interest him; time spent with him, talking, soothing; trying to take a little rest; hurrying down the aisle every time the noise level from the Italians reaches an unacceptable level. 'Si! Si!' they say accommodatingly, nodding sympathetically in Eric's direction. Their ebullience re-surfaces quickly, but they try their best to control it. Eric is restless and dispirited for the first time. He looks like a sixteenth-century doge these days because he did not trust the barber in Venice. Quite distinguished, but a little unfamiliar. It is impossible to cheer him up, but occasionally a delicacy from up front raises a little interest. We have a long, long way to go. Like Dr Busetto I feel like saying to him, 'Mr Phillips! Mr Phillips! You must stay well!'

Something within this noisy machine is separating us more surely than anything that has happened so far. In his restlessness he flings his good arm over the curtain rail and lies on his side. Back to the foetal position of all those weeks ago before he was wheeled into Intensive Care. He does this quite often and is groaning loudly. He is restless. Jonathan, after one of his visits to him says, 'I'm getting worried about the passengers. They'll think we're transporting a crazed orang-utan!'

At Bangkok the Italians depart for good, the plane empties, and the four of us in our party who are mobile go and get a breath of hot, steamy air from the gangway. We watch the plane being cleaned, we tell Eric that the next landing will be Sydney. Nothing seems to reach him. He is lost in his own hell and it is down solely to his endurance and determination now. He is doing it alone. Meanwhile, Sylvia takes advantage of the stop to perform a few nursing duties to make him more comfortable. He submits.

Our new captain pays his respects, but is unsure whether Jonathan will be still able to sit with me. Jonathan resigns himself and settles back with the others, and I close my eyes again but do not even expect sleep.

I had imagined that the first sight of Australia

would be overpoweringly emotional. I now know that deep emotion is quite unpredictable. What you think will happen seldom does. What you are not expecting devours you. I merely note that we have arrived somewhere special and hurry to tell Eric. I push his blind back. 'Look! Look!' I say. 'We're over Australia!' Not even a turn of his head. 'I couldn't give a stuff.' His reaction matches mine obviously, but his expressing of it is surprising. I am the user of coarse language in our duo – not him. At least in public. He is very down, and I am desperately worried. 'Michael. Can he have a vodka?' 'I don't see why not.' And Michael disappears, re-appearing swiftly, glass in hand. It is my belief that the vodka was in a very real sense life-saving. Certainly, he never became as low again, and was much quieter.

The flight will not ever end . . .

> Wedding-Guest! This soul hath been
> Alone on a wide wide sea:
> So lonely 'twas, that God himself
> Scarce seemed there to be.

. . . it will end though, it will end. We sorely troubled souls have, against the odds, made our escape from the Serene City. All will be well.

Soon we shall hear the cry, 'Land ahead! Land ahead!'

The last book I packed before leaving Venice was *A Guide to Paintings in Original Settings: VENICE,* by Terisio Pignatti. I flicked through it briefly, there in the apartment, with some sense of irony about all the words it had not been necessary to digest, all the illustrations destined to remain just that. I stopped at the section Sestiere of San Marco. The first illustration was my Madonna and Child, the only attribution, Byzantine artist (twelfth century). I read that this was the oldest painting in all Venetian art, and that she was brought back from Constantinople by invading Crusaders after the sack of that city. She is known as the Bringer of Victory.

She hangs on my bedroom wall.

Part Two

Love is as mighty as death,
Passion as fierce as the grave;
Its flames are a blazing fire.
Deep waters cannot quench love,
No flood can sweep it away.

Song of Songs
Book of Solomon

We landed at Sydney airport on the evening of Anzac Day. An ambulance was waiting, and Jonathan travelled in it with Michael and Eric. I was met on the plane by an Alitalia representative who assured me of a trouble-free exit through Customs and a swift release through the sliding doors, through the waiting friends and relatives, straight into the arms of 'your family who anxiously await your return'. I smiled weakly and gratefully, and we made our way to the carousel, where my escort and I positioned ourselves perfectly to snatch my bag and Jonathan's.

And the bags began their graceful minuet ...

One or two social phrases floated to the surface as we waited ... and waited ... and I began thinking, If we are not out of here soon I shall be joining Eric in the ambulance. Smiling the while. People joyously or morosely dragged their bags off, children got in the way; people were tetchy or excited or anxious – or all three at once – but what they all did, sooner or later, was *move on*. Sylvia, having collected *her* bag, was about to move on, too. She was by then aware that the taxi situation was not going to be ideal at this airport and was none too pleased. I thanked her and wished her a happy stay in Sydney, but feared, even as the words were forming, that Hull held greater satisfactions.

The throngs had thinned and my escort had examined every piece of luggage, without success. My smile was now so fixed, my general feeling so detached, so unreal, so hazy – a complete sense of absence in other words – that, like Mr Pyecroft, I felt I, too, might float off, up, up to the ceiling, drifting round and round, lazily, lazily – like the dangerously few pieces of luggage still left on the carousel.

Finally, just two bags remained. My kind escort checked and re-checked and assured me that they were definitely not mine.

'It is the wrong name, Mrs Phillips,' he said, in his soft Italian way.

Idly curious . . .

'What name would be on them, I wonder?'

He checked, humouring me.

The name on the two bags was unmistakably Arabic . . . Islamic . . . Bedouin. A romantic name. A name from the great deserts of the world; from the oases, the caravans, the camel routes and the mirages; from the rich and costly tents with their embroidered cushions, their antique rugs, their mystery, their enticement . . . and it was a name that at that moment I hated! It was Sylvia's name, because Sylvia, of course, had been with Jonathan when the luggage – every goddamned piece of it – had been booked all the way to Sydney, all the long, long way to Sydney from Venice. In the confusion of the departure, every piece carried her exotic name. Thus, in Sydney, did I wait. Venice's lion had given a parting flick of his tail.

My charming escort led me, the last one from the flight, through the solid doors that open and close with such finality, through still milling friends and relations, past them all, to three forlorn young women – Anna, Jane and Lisa – who had given up all hope of ever seeing me again. My escort gravely bade me farewell and we headed towards two cars, one of which Jane drove to the hospital to collect Jonathan; the other, mine ... my blissful carriage home ...

The ambulance drive had not been without a flick of the lion's tail either. At last on their way – through the gates and heading north – suddenly Michael noticed the absence of the two Eskies of blood and plasma. The ambulance made a careful U turn and they sped back to the airport, only to find the gate locked. My son, not unused to the ways of Security, managed to attract the attention of the requisite holder of the key, the gates swung open, and the ambulance returned to the by now quiet plane. Inside, someone was whistling happily, wielding mop and broom, not at all disturbed by two unattended Eskies – ever hopeful, perhaps, that they contained caviar and champagne.

The Eskies joined them in the ambulance, and my husband was at last on *his* way – his future now able to be assessed in conditions that would be familiar, comforting, and, above all, free of the nightmarish uncertainties of the Venetian sojourn. He could begin to re-assert some control over his life.

Anna, Jane, Jonathan and I came together again in an hour or two. Lisa took a snap that is testament to our weariness and strain, we supped briefly, and then bed, my own – for now unshared – beckoned. Sleep was allowed to take over. The moments before sleep I had mostly heretofore found deliciously satisfying – a gentle easing into unconsciousness, anxieties on hold, a brief wandering through the events of the day, a glance at the events of the next; and whether those events seemed challenging, difficult, delightful, or alarming, they were mostly more or less under my control. Some sense of order prevailed. I was not rudderless – even at the most difficult of times. In the seconds – minutes – before sleep on Anzac night, I was aware that the immediate past had entered every cell of my body to the exclusion of all else. No other past existed. The future was wrapped around a nucleus called Eric. Additions to that nucleus were yet to be revealed, but any future outside it was unimaginable. What I would become from now on was dependent on just the one chain reaction.

And so, as I had predicted from a great and unassailable high just a few short months before, Venice did indeed show me – not what lay ahead, how could she? – but surely and inescapably, what my path was.

Sunday at the hospital. The Sydney Adventist Hospital is a large private hospital run by the Seventh Day Adventists at Wahroonga. It has a considerable acreage surrounding it, which early in its history, when The San was little more than a large two-storeyed house, was given over to vegetable gardens and herds of cows – for milk only in this strictly vegetarian community. Still strictly vegetarian for the followers, but today meat, if required, is available to the rest of us.

It seemed a country retreat in those days, but now fields have given way to carparks, there is a school, and the houses of the Adventist community radiate for more than a kilometre or two. It is a fine hospital with a high reputation, excellent staff and the most modern equipment. Eric was familiar with it, not through any personal experience, but through visiting me on and off over the years.

Directly opposite the entrance doors are the lifts, and on that first Sunday, Jane and I made our way to the tenth floor, turned left and went into his room, Anna already there. We were like children at a party, exclaiming at the comfort of the room, the view over the treetops, the pristine state of everything, including, oh joy, the bathroom, and delighting, above all, in the smiles on the faces of every nurse who popped in. The overall impression was of a somewhat subdued party where the guest of honour just happened to be in bed – and asleep. There were even two Eskies on the dressing table ...

Occasionally, Eric surfaced. He was unmistakably bearded now and looked more and more like one of the early Venetian doges. His eyes were relaxed at last and I hoped in his few conscious moments he was in a fine state of self-congratulation. Every prideful moment had he earned in spades.

'Oh, darling! This is heaven!' – over and over ...

The girls and I wandered in and out, went to the

café downstairs for healthful, tasteless sandwiches, and, after Venice, undrinkable coffee, but who cared! Dr Jean-Pierre Halpert, the associate neurologist, had by then examined him. We met briefly. He indicated physiotherapy would start very soon because those first few weeks after the stroke had been lost. There were to be tests, of course, there were to be scans and x-rays, the reports from Venice would be picked over – there was, in short, much to be done; but for this first Sunday we all were simply adjusting and revelling in, aside from anything else, the blissful ease of communication.

On the Monday Eric's haematologist examined him, and I met Geoffrey Herkes, the neurologist, and Michael Dodd, the lung specialist. Geoff Herkes was kind, supportive and enormously encouraging to Eric once his attempts at physiotherapy began. He was always our first line of contact. Some of the results would be available the next night, and I made an appointment with him for seven o'clock.

Our house is solace and sanctuary. I walk through its rooms feeling luxurious, pampered, by virtue of space, objects, and nearly forty-one years of accumulated history. Our history. It wraps itself around me gently and, even in his absence, I am not lonely. I want him here again, but I am not desolate without him, certain now that he is on the right track and all will be well. The exodus from Venice, the highly dangerous exodus, is behind us. Outside, the garden, as usual, is its lovely tangle and the cat, by now returned, explores with me, never far from my side, making me aware, at every turn, that she will not appreciate separation again.

The phone rang and rang, but visits were postponed for just a day or two to allow for recovery from the journey. *I* knew how close Eric had come to letting go. He needed to gather himself again. I pictured, or tried to picture, our future, which for the moment was inescapably bound up with the degree of paralysis he would be left with from the stroke. It was strange to recall how little the stroke had featured in our thinking in Venice. Here, Geoff Herkes was making it a priority. Eric was to be turned towards rehabilitation. We could accommodate to anything, I felt. He and I had already glimpsed wonders and horrors. Because of them, we had discovered a closeness – different, more intense – than any experienced before, deeper, even, than at the height of our first passionate discoveries.

Tuesday evening at the appointed time, Eric was sitting up in bed. His room was already full of flowers, messages, and the beginnings of a large collection of artwork by his grandchildren. He was already stronger. He smiled, greeting with his well-honed sentences. Delightfully odd words would appear at times. We loved them. Geoff Herkes was persuading him to try to exercise the paralysed right leg as he lay there. He discussed speech therapy with him and arrangements for this were to be put in train.

And then Geoff rose to his feet. I walked with him to the door, sickeningly aware, as in Venice, that we had not reached the subtext yet. We went into the corridor.

Eric's lung had been x-rayed, the three specialists, having examined the results from Venice, needing to confirm what was obviously at the forefront of their thinking. So …

'Eric has lung cancer,' he said. 'An aggressive cancer. It is already in the lymph nodes.'

I digested this for a moment or two, as from the bed behind the closed door came an imperious, 'Yes! Yes!'

I knew my husband would not be patient for long.

'How long do you think?' I was surprised that a voice had emerged.

'Twelve, perhaps fifteen months.'

'Oh ... fuck ...' It was just an exhalation.

And quietly back from him, 'This is the greatest life crisis you will ever face.' I, nodding, nodding ...

'Yes!! Yes!!' even more imperiously from the room.

'I'll have to go to him. He'll want to know.'

There would be a consultation the next day with the lung specialist.

'Yes,' I said.

I went in to him. The eyes meeting mine were steely and there was not going to be any escape. Not that there was any question of escape.

'You want to know?'

'Yes!'

So I told him. He wanted to know everything. So I told him.

'Fifteen months?'

There might have been a few tears, but I do not think so. What I do remember is his clear comprehension and total acceptance ... and, tangibly, the cord between us tightening, tightening ...

Actually, at the time, we were pretty cool, as I recall. Real cool cats.

Why was I so devastated by this news? I had, after all, faced, in Venice, the almost certain prospect of his death. He had jousted with it on the plane ride home. I had been living with his dying for over three weeks. I suppose that when we got back, I thought we had won. The blood condition would be sorted out, the stroke was being dealt with, there was no reason why with care and the most modern of techniques, and with the time now available to apply them, he should not gradually be at a point where he would return and live – a very different but still satisfying life. I simply had not thought of cancer – at the conscious level. If I had, I would not have been thinking of such a devastatingly rapid cancer.

Fifteen months – when I was looking forward to years – seemed unthinkable.

There was no question of operating. He was too ill, and attached as the cancer already was to the lymph nodes it would have been a pointless exercise. There was never any question of chemotherapy, either, this particular cancer – a squamous cell carcinoma – not being responsive to the process.

His blood was now doing the opposite from its dangerous behaviour in Venice. It was clotting. A major problem, which required vigilant monitoring and careful adjustments. His blood was sent off for *particular* analysis. When the result came back, ten days later, Eric was discovered to be among the less than one per cent of the population with an auto-immune disorder called antiphospholipid syndrome. The majority of those with this syndrome, and no underlying cancer, are walking around, their condition under control with medication. Eric's was almost out of control and required a drip of the drug Heparin, which controls clotting. His highly unstable and unpredictable blood was another reason, of course, that he would not have survived surgery ...

He had started to experience some pain in his right wrist, too, so a rheumatologist was invited to join the team. No one wanted to do a bone scan in those early days because there were too many other scans and tests, all of them higher priorities. One required a visit to Northside Imaging for an MRI machine that would closely examine the shadow in his brain, a shadow that may or may not have been caused by the stroke. The result showed it was indeed connected with the stroke and excluded the possibility of a secondary cancer in that site. With all this exhausting activity, any investigation of the painful right wrist was put on hold. Michael Dodd, the lung specialist, saw Eric and me together and was not backward in explaining the aggressive nature of the cancer.

As each piece of information was received, it was passed on to Eric. He quietly took it all on board.

And all his grandchildren came to see him ...

I remember vividly at the funeral of a friend the year before how moved Eric had been by the contribution made by our friend's grandchildren. Their loss was palpable. At the same time, their celebration of their grandfather was eloquent and moving. I remember Eric saying as we left, 'I have to make more time, they're closer to Jim than ours are to me. I'm missing out.'

'*I wish,*' he had said.

And, ironically, as with Anna and her desire to get to Venice, the events there made it directly possible for *his* wish, too, to be granted. His grand-children were in and out of his room, clambering all over his bed, and their continuing delight in each other was one of the great plusses of this journey.

In the midst of all this, one major professional commitment lay ahead for me, and was occupying all thought that was not exclusively bound up in him. I was scheduled to start rehearsals of Edward Albee's *A Delicate Balance* in just under two months. Eric knew this, and our first week home proceeded with the knowledge that this, somehow or other, would indeed be happening. I think I longed for him to ask me to pull out. Pulling out was something I had never even contemplated before, despite extreme difficulties at times. Every fibre of my body worked against any such decision, the moral imperative up till now pointing in one direction only. 'You've signed for it! Do it!' I, therefore, anticipated I would be 'doing' it. I dreaded the prospect, but was arrogant enough to believe I could make it all work. The children knew the play was looming, but everyone avoided talking about it. It just hung there in the air.

One week after we arrived home, Anna and I went to a play at NIDA. It was performed without an interval and lasted just ninety minutes. After fifteen minutes, despite the brisk delightfulness of performance and production, I was so exhausted, so barely able to stay in my seat, that the deeply troubling matter hanging over all our heads resolved itself. Driving me back to Wahroonga afterwards, Anna blurted out, 'You just can't do the play. Please don't!'

The first time it had been brought into the open.

'I'm not, I'm not ... there's just no *energy* for anything else ...'

Nor any desire, I could have added.

At the hospital I told Eric.

'I'm so glad. I'm *so glad!*' And then he was crying.

'Why on earth didn't you say something? You know how I've been agonizing over it!'

'No! It had to come from you!'

When did the roller coaster start? At what point did I slip into the seat, grip the bar, shut eyes tightly – and from that moment never again know for sure whether we were up or down?

On the one hand, physiotherapy proceeded – if not exactly swiftly – then with determination on Eric's part. Geoff Herkes was always way, way up in enthusiasm and encouragement for Eric's efforts. The slightest twitch in the paralysed right leg resulted in such delight from his neurologist that we would all feel a major hurdle had been cleared and, any day now, any bright late autumn day, he and I would be waltzing again …

Eric, it must be remembered, had been unable to move without help since the morning of April 6, when the stroke had occurred. He had the use of his left side, but he had not been out of bed since that moment. We were now into May, and he was only just beginning tiny exercises, working up to sitting on the side of the bed. Every minuscule advance caused delight, not only to the patient, but throughout Floor 10, it seemed. I remember the great and glorious day a nurse called out as I was walking to his room, 'Mrs Phillips! Mrs Phillips! He stood today! He stood!'

Her joy outstripping mine.

Eric's joy earlier had way outstripped ours ... 'Where's Mum? Where's Mum?' he had said to Anna. 'I have special news!' And then he was crying ... 'It is the first time I have seen out a window in six weeks.'

He had also started speech therapy, but much of the tediousness of this process irritated him. He persevered, but his intelligence seemed to get in the way of progress here – a not uncommon reaction, I imagine. When the brain has outstripped the kindergarten requirements of learning to speak properly again, frustrations need to be worked at with infinite tact. It was difficult to persuade him to practise, particularly as he and I had no difficulty communicating. A bad attitude this, and not to be encouraged.

So work proceeded and our goal, which I never doubted, was for him to be back home in three months, just about the time I would be re-rehearsing for the Sydney season of *A Little Night Music*. It would be a hairy time, this, but on the up swing of the roller coaster, it seemed a pushover!

Eric's spirits, too, were mostly buoyant. This helped me to be optimistic. I was still anxious, but we did seem to be making progress – slowly, yes, but with great good cheer – towards a time when we would be peacefully together, richly together, at home. So what if it *was* only one year – that year was going to be memorable.

I had visions of gatherings where *he* would be the centre – in or out of a wheelchair. I would create a salon for him where there would be amusing conversation, music, laughter, gentle intimacies, ribaldry and gossip. He would be surrounded and pampered. The food and wine would be exquisite; we would have a fine time – as the garden moved through the seasons ...

As ever, off on my daydream ...

Just the same – who can say when someone will

die? It could be longer, much longer, than twelve months. His iron determination could succeed in confounding them all. Kirrily, for one, refused to believe Eric could be dying. In many ways the most extraordinary man in her life, she invested him with an immortality that was both seductive and, as time progressed, dangerous. But her unassailable conviction was heady and persuasive when the roller coaster was poised way, way up.

Just occasionally, there would be a puzzling jolt. Why, for instance, did one of the senior sisters take me aside one day? Why was she compelled to tell me that she knew what I was going through? Her own husband had died the year before from secondary cancers – the primary source never discovered – and she seemed concerned about me and determined that I should take care of myself and in some way – what? Be prepared? And yes, I could put all this down to the fact that Eric's time *was* limited, but the urgency of this conversation, the compassion, seemed to put the end much closer – imminent, even. On the one hand, we were doing everything to ready him for a return home as soon as possible; on the other hand – something else was slithering alongside. There was a serpent here – some subterranean knowledge I was not as yet privy to …

And the night nurse, a man highly experienced in oncology, sometimes seemed as if he were attending to a dying man …

These moments passed. I felt I must have an imagination too highly attuned – unreliably attuned – and soon the roller coaster would head upwards again …

Routines developed as they always do – to preserve equilibrium, sanity. Anna had returned to her family, maintaining twice-weekly visits; Jonathan returned to New Guinea for two weeks; Jane, close at hand, was able to visit easily.

Eric was receiving other visitors by now, and enjoying them. Some, not all, of our staff visited him. Some felt they could not bear to see him as he now was, considering their last view of him had been of a vigorous, forward-thinking employer. The businesses continued for the time being without him, though he was kept up to date, and was still firmly committed to moving one of our galleries to another location. I let that one pass.

I would go to The San at least twice a day. I began reading to him, and this he enjoyed so much that it became a continuing activity. We started with a tale of the search for the provenance of a painting, *A Small Unsigned Painting* by Stephen Scheding. It mentioned many people Eric knew, or knew of, and the journey to prove whether or not the painting was a Lloyd Rees delighted him. While always appreciating visitors and responding to them warmly, his chief joy was to have me to himself, particularly as we wove our way through the intricacies of the Lloyd Rees mystery. I read the newspaper to him, too. He did not have much energy for this himself, nor, indeed, for television, but we did set him up with music, which had always been a shared pleasure.

The most surprising development was that Eric, with little experience in these matters, was metamorphosing into the sort of patient who actually enjoys hospital routine. This astounded me, for he had never given any indication in his rare bouts with minor ailments that he had any patience whatever. Deprived of the day-to-day sociability that went with his working life, he seemed happy to substitute his present routine for what he no longer had. He became an ideal patient, in other words, and certainly all the staff seemed very attached to him. His huge delight, for instance, whenever he had a bath in the extraordinary portable contraption used for the not so mobile, was infectious. It was a performance and, given the opportunity, he never tired of stepping into the spotlight.

The only cloud on the horizon was the continuing saga of the hearing aid. In the course of his stay it was returned to the manufacturers at least half a dozen times. Kirrily would collect it, rush it to their premises in George Street; it would be adjusted within an inch of its life and then returned, kindly, by courier. The drama would subside for a day or two – and then we would be at it again. I have never hated anything quite so much. On one memorable occasion, after the usual tantrum from my beloved, I stood by the window tossing it in my hand. He knew me well enough to know that limits had been reached. I ached to hurl it to the furthest reaches of Wahroonga –

all two thousand dollars' worth. There was a stand-off for a short time, and then a grudging apology – one of the very few received by me during our marriage. We kissed and made up, and from that moment the hearing aid miraculously lost its malevolence.

One day around about this time Eric tired of being a doge. I walked in, the beard had disappeared, and he was instantly closer to the man I had lived with for all those years. Possibly just a coincidence that the hearing aid improved the minute the beard disappeared.

Eric was never short of women visitors who were prepared to give him a manicure or moustache trim – mostly younger women, which added to the impression, at times, of an Eastern potentate receiving the tender attentions of the harem. We had moved from Venice to something altogether more exotic. All of which he accepted as his due. Kirrily and Lisa, I seem to remember, ministered particularly in these areas. I just knew it was not on my list.

Each day I drove to The San, I drove back from The San and I drove to The San. I never complained.

I had a car. After Venice I was living a life of luxury – though living it a touch too impatiently at times in my race to get to the bedside. Once, cutting a bit rudely in front of a dilatory driver, I was roundly tooted:

'If you have a beloved who has an aggressive lung cancer, a stroke, *and* a chaotic antiphospholipid syndrome,' I snarled, 'feel at liberty to toot, not otherwise!'

A set of conditions not often likely to be met, I felt.

Eric was able to sit in a chair now for a time each day – a great leap forward. He was busy with the speech therapy and the physiotherapy and was applying all the singleness of purpose to these two tasks – despite his reservations about the efficacy of the former – that had made him such a successful businessman and entrepreneur. Progress every day, and it was thrilling. He was still on a Heparin drip, and was now taking Warfarin orally, to further impair his clotting. This aside, he was undoubtedly making progress. His three specialists were in constant attendance. We all seemed to be waiting – though, looking back, I am not sure that we were all waiting for the same thing. I was waiting to get him home as soon as possible. I was not thinking too much about how it would be managed. I desired it, simple as that, and if occasionally, out of the corner of my eye, I was aware of something sliding across his hospital room, I avoided looking at it.

Eric's bed was of the Rolls Royce variety. It was delivered with a degree of ceremony a week or two after his arrival, and was designed to make those needing to spend most of their days horizontal as comfortable as humanly possible. It tilted in every direction and seemed to have a deliciously wavy contour that was inviting in the extreme. I would have been in there with him in a flash during exhausting days and nights, but was thwarted by drips and attachments. The bed succeeded admirably in discouraging any hint of bedsores.

Three weeks or so after Eric's admission, the decision was taken to remove the Heparin drip. This step had to be taken at some stage or Eric would never be leaving hospital. The Heparin would now be delivered through direct injection under the skin – a convenient method that would presumably be able to be self-administered at some later stage.

Within twenty-four hours of the removal of the drip his right leg blew up in a massive clot that extended from toes to groin. At any time now, a smaller clot could fatally break away. Somehow it did not ...

The Heparin returned to the drip and we took more than a step or two backwards.

But still the physiotherapy progressed apace; still the determination of the patient showed no signs of wavering. The newspapers were read to him and commented upon – he found much to irritate him – and the story of the hunt for the Lloyd Rees provenance drew to a disappointing conclusion, or so we felt; family were around at week-ends; so many delights for him – all for the asking. Our factory manager had called to see him, and the number two framer. Many of our staff. Those who did were all shaken by the change that had occurred in just five or six short weeks. A crack was opening.

Except for Kirrily – still buoyant, optimistic – sure of his almost superhuman powers ...

National Sorry Day was 26 May 1998. It began with a ceremony at Government House, to which I had been invited along with others who had been closely associated with the process of Reconciliation with the first inhabitants of our island continent. It was a moving and warm occasion and a lovely, if brief, break for me with many friends – black and white. I stayed as long as I could, and then made the long journey to Wahroonga, with a sense of optimism that in these vital areas we at last seemed to be making a modicum of progress. I was hurrying to report to Eric on the ceremony.

We had an appointment first with Dr Stephen Buckley, Consultant in Rehabilitation Medicine from the Mount Wilga Rehabilitation Hospital at Hornsby. It was planned that Eric would be going there just as soon as possible because, once stable and strong enough, there would be no further reason for him to be taking up a precious bed at the Adventist Hospital. Leaving the security of The San was not something I was looking forward to, but I knew it was not only inevitable, but desirable. Stephen Buckley met Eric and me, gave us details of how Mount

Wilga operated – what its aims were – and confidently predicted that Eric's attitude made him an ideal person to benefit from their methods and all they had to offer. After he left, I told Eric about the Sorry Day ceremony, we read, we talked, we sat quietly. I drove home, coped with the necessary domestic details, did some shopping, returned for yet another meeting, this time with Geoff Herkes. Eric had at last had his bone scan, and the result would be available.

Geoff and I had one of our corridor meetings.

The result was devastating. Metastases of the cancer to the wrist, the ribs, the vertebrae.

I thanked him and returned to the bedside.

Eric was waiting. Eric was told. Eric shrugged.

Next day, Jane and I were scheduled for a meeting with his specialists.

We were all ushered into a tiny office at seven that evening. Cramped, as I recall, not enough room for chairs, but we were happier standing, bumping into one another as x-rays were pored over, held up to the light, explained, discussed, compared, argued over. All academic, really, but Michael Dodd seemed to be cutting through the discussions, almost despairingly at times. For the first time I warmed to him. I sensed he was telling it like it was – no frills here, no dressing up ... no softening obligato ... this was plainsong ... no colour ... film noir ...

... life noir ...

Eric's lung specialist even seemed to be arguing about the antiphospholipid findings – not their accuracy, but that none of it really mattered too much in the face of this all-conquering carcinoma. That, indeed, the cancer could have been prime *cause* of the syndrome. The cancer that, upon further examination of the slides, had shown itself to be not squamous cell as first reported, but 'large cell undifferentiated'. At this remove, I do not care too much. Chicken and egg. But the concern and disappointment for all three specialists – and the frustration – well, what else does one say. It comes with the job. One thing they could offer – palliative radiotherapy to alleviate pain.

Silence for a moment.

And at the top of a filing cabinet the confident serpent was not even bothering to conceal himself.

We would be going ahead with Mount Wilga as planned because, still, there is no way of predicting just how long these – occasions – take. Prediction is impossible. There is an ancient process at work that resolutely defies all the experts, all the knowledge – something primitive, atavistic; each journey uniquely individual – which is the marvel of it.

Right now, Eric was alive.

Throughout our life together, Eric had approached all problems with the clearest of heads, the coolest of eyes. Problems were there to be solved. He brought a mathematical detachment to the task, which mostly ran rings round my more emotional and instinctive approach. His present problem he refined back to the simple business of making himself strong enough to live his life to the full, however restrictive and undesirable that 'full' might seem to others. Not to him. Put simply, Eric still had things to do.

Thus, we readied ourselves for Mount Wilga. We knew that his neurologist would be on call at all times, likewise his haematologist, but basically he would now be in the hands of Stephen Buckley.

Before he left the Adventist Hospital, Eric was given a blood transfusion. He was no longer on the Heparin by drip but as an injected form, which seemed to be controlling the clotting tendency. This, of course, was what made the transfer possible. His blood would continue to be closely monitored – any emergencies able to be swiftly dealt with.

Eric left The San on June 2, Jane and I following his stretcher as he left his room and was wheeled towards the lift. As he passed the nursing station his booming voice called out 'Good-bye!' towards the three who were working there – three of his new friends. He raised his good arm triumphantly, and it was as well he did for it hid his eyes, which were suddenly full of tears –

Wish me luck as you wave me good-bye
Cheerio here I go on my way . . .

Eric had donned his straw boater again, set it at a jaunty angle – there was no place for tears!

And as he was pushed into the lift, he could just

hear, coming back to him in snappy three-part harmony –

> We don't want to lose you
> But we know you have to go ...

Jane went with him in the ambulance. I followed behind in my car, keeping close. This was our first visit to Mount Wilga – I did not want to lose them. We went through Hornsby following the old Pacific Highway. In the ambulance, Eric was focused on all the familiar landmarks – totally aware, absorbed.

After a few kilometres, we made a turn or two left, towards a gully, and there we were. I parked; watched Eric being carried into his new dwelling, hoping, hoping he would be happy here.

To our delight we found that Stephen Buckley had turned a double room into a single. This meant that Eric had plenty of space and a view straight out to the garden, which would prove a godsend. From his window we could see the large two-storey house next door that had once belonged to Mount Wilga, but was now owned by a religious group who went about their affairs quietly. The paths through the garden still connected, so it would be possible to wheel Eric right around the old house and back again. There was a gazebo outside his window, which we would make good use of.

Jane and I were welcomed and we proceeded to a conference room where a charming sister called Fiona took all details – a little nervously, excitedly. We were advised of the facilities, taken through the routines, given some reading matter. We were shown the gymnasium and swimming pool, and advised how the day's programme for Eric would operate. There was a whiteboard in his room, which would indicate his schedule for the day, and there would be a porter to transport him to the relevant activities. The slightly alarming discipline of the place did not disturb Eric at all. He could not wait to begin.

Earlier, we had set him up with track suits, tops that were easy to get in and out of and soft shoes that were strong enough for him to walk in. All utterly absurd it seemed to me on the down swing of the roller coaster, but for Eric a new, highly exciting and challenging adventure was beginning.

For one thing, he would be dressing for the first time in more than two months. Dressing with assistance was an essential part of his 'training' here.

There was a dining room where he would be wheeled for the main meal of the day, which, if so desired, I could participate in. I didn't so desire!

A shared bathroom, too, but this one presenting none of the difficulties of Venice.

There would be three main areas of 'work' for Eric –

Physiotherapy: His aim here would be to perform tasks such as 'bed mobility, moving from lying/sitting/standing, balance, walking, stairs, reaching, grasping and manipulation of everyday objects, flexibility and fitness'.
Speech Pathology: where he would seek 'clarity of speech, voice quality, conversational skills, fluency, understanding and use of speech, reading, spelling and writing, swallowing'.
Occupational Therapy: where he would be retrained, where necessary, to 'maximise independent functioning' in the business of self-care, home management

skills, work-related activities, leisure skills, driving – I was eagerly looking forward to the day when I might be a passenger – plus upper limb and hand function retraining where the tasks would be reaching for everyday objects, using a knife and fork, handwriting and the undoing and doing up of his buttons.

He, and we, would also have the use of a social worker, if required.

Jane and I finished our business with Fiona and visited Eric – ensconced in bed and certainly smiling. Looking at the fragile body, aware of some of the things going on *inside* that body, I might wonder for just a moment what on earth this was all about. Only for a moment, though, as I became, now and in the days ahead, ever more aware of Eric's supreme will – of such a high order that at times the magical word 'remission' swam in a bubble above him and you could believe anything was possible.

Eric's 'contact person' at Mount Wilga was Paula Peres, his physiotherapist. Medical needs would be in the hands of Dr Ragupathy Rengathan – universally known as Dr Ragu due to the distressing inability of most Australians to get their tongues and lips around unfamiliar combinations of consonants and vowels.

I quickly became familiar with all aspects of Mount Wilga. I knew where coffee could be made – well, instant, but by now not going to be spurned by me when nerve ends were screaming. Bread, too, was in a cupboard for toasting, and sometimes unexpected goodies in the fridge. I do hope they were for general consumption. At times one might be at a health farm. Incredibly busy, always, people being escorted or wheeled to various strenuous activities.

A slightly bizarre touch was added by the presence, on the other side of the carpark fence, of a shooting range. A red flag would go up and suddenly shots would be heard. I felt I should be scanning the sky for falling ducks, but this, of course, was serious, disciplined shooting at stationary targets. Nothing frivolous. The wildlife was safe. Sometimes, though, as one emerged from one's car, a tendency to drop to the ground as the firing started could cause embarrassment.

My visits would be planned around the evening's

information on the whiteboard in Eric's room. If he had an early session with the physiotherapist or speech therapist, I would tend to arrive afterwards.

Whatever time I arrived in the morning, it was never early enough for Eric. There would be a phone call, which sometimes he could manage unaided, and the voice, getting a little hoarse these days, would strike straight to the heart, so that the few up till then essential chores at the home base quickly receded in importance.

The face lighting up as I entered his room was still gold in a creek bed ...

I was now reading Barry Humphries' *More Please,* which proved a major hit, not only with him, but with any other members of the family who might be there. I had a veritable reading group, and the book choice could not have been bettered. Cleaners lingered ... and all, as I told Barry on a plane much later, engrossed, entertained, giggling.

Hullo, girls and boys! I'm going to tell you a story about a wolf! You'll like that, won't you? Grrr!!! A very clever wolf who sometimes frightened the other animals ...

Lovely looking out his window, too, as autumn passed and winter began. Birds everywhere. Eric urged me to look out at the chooks one day.

'What are you talking about? There are no chooks there.'

'Yes! Yes! Look at that one getting under the ... thing!'

A galah pushed under the hedge into the next garden.

'A galah!' I said.

'That's right! A carrot! They're in the tree, too.'

I began to attend the physiotherapy sessions, conducted by his 'contact', Paula Peres. Eric developed a highly flirtatious relationship with Paula. She had his measure completely and they had a rapport that was delightful to watch. This rapport, as much as his strong will, was responsible for his wonderful progress, given everything that was stacked against him. I sat there one day and watched him walk – with support close at hand and ready to spring if necessary – from one end of the gym to the other. Focus, focus, focus. But tired, so tired, when he had finished. He was managing all the required tasks with eating, and progressing with showering. I could feel I was watching the odds change – for just a while. He was brilliant.

Geoff Herkes suggested that we should try to get Eric home for a day. We should try to give him one or two memorable days.

One or two ... the odds lengthened again. Up and down on the roller coaster ...

So we did just that. We brought him home. We planned our first great feast day for the Monday of the Queen's Birthday week-end. Jonathan was back from New Guinea – the timing was perfect.

We prepared very carefully, and Jonathan went to Mount Wilga on the Saturday to be instructed in how to transport him safely, and we got all the shopping done, and everyone had a job to do, and we planned a menu that was suitable and beautiful and we looked for his best bottles of wine. All over that week-end we prepared for our gathering.

JUNE 8: A fine, cold day. The camellias are out. I am up early getting the house ready. I have decided we will lunch in the drawing room because it will save manoeuvring the wheelchair into the dining room. Less tiring for him. He can sit on the front verandah for awhile if he wants to, and from there it will be just one step up and an easy turn into my sanctuary. We will set up a small table at which he and I will sit, and two or three others at a time can take it in turns to join us. For the rest, plates on knees. The children can eat on the side verandah – they prefer to anyway – the younger ones playing their games, making their 'cubbies' under the table. They will come and go, of course, but when we are eating we will keep it as peaceful as possible for him.

I go into the garden to pick camellias, the cat, already aware that today will be different, accompanying me. She has missed Eric – their night-time routine of 'You can jump onto my lap *now*' still being searched for, his chair having to provide an unsatisfactory substitute.

I imagine him, too, preparing at Mount Wilga. He will have breakfasted in bed. Then he will be helped to the bathroom where he will resolutely tackle his tasks, under supervision; then he will dress – he will be helping them help him, determined and focused as ever. He will be made comfortable in the chair, while he waits for Jonathan to come and help transfer him to the wheelchair, to the car. I imagine how impatient he will be, and more than a little nervous ...

I find I am nervous, too, but at the same time very excited – rather like a bride.

Absurd.

The house looks wonderful now.

Everyone beginning to arrive with their platters and bowls of food ... *everyone*, nervous, it seems, except the children – they are just excited, though occasionally the older ones pause, fall silent for a moment or two, caught between innocence and something else not yet fully understood ...

Jonathan and Lisa arrive with marlin from the fish markets. The required bottles of Grange and Tyrell's Dry Red are dug out, set aside.

Then, at last, it is time for Jonathan to leave for Mount Wilga. In his absence we attend to the finishing touches – and finally there is absolutely nothing left to do, but wait.

When the car returns we are all gathered on the front verandah. We are a family portrait – a little too stiff. Phillip goes to help unload the cargo. I find I am frozen, eyes fixed on the gate ... there is more waiting ... it is taking an eternity to get him out and into the wheelchair, but at last the wheelchair is glimpsed. Now, they are manoeuvring it through the gate.

No longer frozen, the tears are streaming down my face, but I am rooted to the spot until one of my daughters hisses, 'Go and meet him!' So I do, and it is terribly hard to embrace anyone properly when they are in a wheelchair and one arm is in a sling. 'Welcome home! Welcome!' is what I stammer, and he is wheeled to the verandah – up the one step. He has not spoken yet at all, but his eyes are saying everything. Now he is looking at the almost bare china pear – a tracery of branches, twigs, a few last leaves.

The wheelchair is turned to face it. He still does not want to speak. He seems to be immersing himself in a garden he has not seen for ten long, bewildering, chaotic weeks. Drowning in it ...

Gradually, we all relax and the day can begin to assume a degree of normality – or can it? Never before has he been here as guest and no matter what tact is used, with what perception and care he is treated, no matter what deference is paid him, nothing alters the fact that for the first time Eric is no longer host in his own domain. Eric, for the time being, is only ... honoured guest.

I keep looking at him ... looking at his face deeply etched with all his hard-won victories ... seeing all too clearly from his fragile demeanour at just what great cost ... But ... having him home, having him actually home again ... how fantastically, unbelievably wonderful! I am overwhelmed with love.

We bring him inside eventually, wheel him to the corner near the fireplace. He holds court. He is quietly patrician. Jonathan brings the bottle of Grange Hermitage for his approval; Phillip the Tyrell's Dry Red. This is a serious moment. There is confirmation from him that the choice is a fine one.

Jonathan commences the cooking – and in a little while Eric is wheeled to the table, the candles are lit, and lunch is served.

I am at his side for the entire lovely meal, occasionally helping, but mostly he manages on his own. The glass has to be placed near his left hand, though he does not drink a great deal – he, one of the great imbibers of wine. The rest of us make up for him. And the conversation flows, the children come and go, grown-ups play musical chairs with the three seats at the oval table, we have the best feast in the world – though, all through that lunch there will be times when someone will drop out of the conversation, one or two who glance out a window and take awhile to return to the moment. I am wholly in the moment throughout the precious hours because I feel if I retreat I may not find my way back …

There is fruit, cheese. He eats slowly. But no one is in a hurry. We sip the coffee, call for more. Tell stories. It is a day that should go on forever. We are hanging onto it, reluctant to let it slip away from us.

But it is not for us to decide anyway, it is the guest's prerogative, and when the guest decides he must leave our table, we rise and say, 'Of course,' and he is escorted to the waiting car.

Everyone runs onto the footpath this time to bid him farewell. We wave and cry, 'Come again, won't you?' as the car makes its turn and slowly disappears ...

... gone, gone, the day has gone ...

The morning after our feast there was something designated a 'family conference' at Mount Wilga. This, Jane, Jonathan and I discovered, was a meeting in Stephen Buckley's office attended by all who had, or might have, dealings with Eric – physiotherapist, occupational therapist, speech therapist, social worker, dietitian.

We met at ten, crowding in, fitting round and about the centre of attention, Eric in his wheelchair, who occupied a corner. A porter had brought him, and would return at the end of the meeting to collect him. Stephen Buckley chaired the meeting, everyone reported on Eric's progress and it was obvious he was being awarded straight 'A's. We were told that as it approached the time for Eric to return home, the occupational therapist – Or was it the social worker? Surely not the speech therapist! – would come and check our house to ascertain the problem areas for a wheelchair, make suggestions as to what simple changes could be made to make life easier. Where a rail or two could be added.

As the meeting proceeded, energetically and with great enthusiasm, as Eric was consulted, nodded, answered questions; as we were urged to support him in all his work, particularly speech and physiotherapy, we could have been attending a meeting whose endgame was fixed and certain and where no doubts whatever were felt or acknowledged by any. The moments of doubt, veering close to scepticism, experienced by me at times, were gradually swamped by the high confidence and strength-through-joy atmosphere of the day – to borrow an erstwhile phrase of Eric's to describe such gatherings – and I found myself caught up in the general bonhomie. It was heady, and I refused to raise my eyes to the picture rail, knowing all too well what could be there, watching. Eric himself was confident and determined. How dared I, in the face of that, allow any doubts to intrude.

So I raised my spirits high. I watched him at his

tasks. I marvelled at his good humour. He still had a low boredom threshold where the foolish and fawning were concerned, but fortunately few of these swam into view at Mount Wilga. All we saw were committed and optimistic people. People who were dealing on a daily basis with the handicapped – either through stroke, trauma or neurological disease – and who managed to instil in nearly all these people a kernel of their own spirit. Looking at Eric, how could I wish it any other way? And, again and again, to counter all negativity (or realism?) on my part that bubble containing the one word 'remission' twinkled above his head. Even knowing all we did about his condition, I do not believe he entertained a doubt for a second that he would not be wheeled, or helped, through our front door for a rich twelve or so months that would be the climax of our forty-one years. As ever throughout our life, he was the one to bolster my flagging spirits and persuade me that anything at all was possible.

But . . . a few days later, Stephen Buckley stopped me in the garden. I had just come away from watching still more miracles under Paula Peres. Stephen told me that he would like to see Eric alone. He asked me pointedly whether or not Eric was aware of his condition.

'Of course!'

'I really can't believe he can know,' he responded, 'how *very* ill he is ...'

'He does,' I said. 'He knows absolutely that his time is limited.'

'... because I can't say where he will be *in five or six weeks' time!*'

No ambivalence, no ambiguity, no indecision, no escape ...

... and the serpent with his subterranean knowledge could now depart the scene. I was initiated.

They must have had their meeting, Eric and Stephen, but there was never any indication from Eric whatsoever that circumstances had changed by so much as a ripple. The waters were calm, we were still sailing serenely. I marvelled at how he seemed to have so surely and instinctively arrived at a state of 'active peace' that, with others, takes many hours of meditation, counselling ... he had entered a special state of grace all by himself ... or was he simply rejecting what he had been told? ... indeed, *had* he been told? I did not ask.

I have a sudden memory of us. We are in the south-western corner of Australia. There is a gale blowing, but we have climbed to the top of the Cape Leeuwin Lighthouse. We force our way outside and I find it thrilling, with him there beside me. We look down, down at the boiling sea, looking at the very place where the Indian and Southern oceans converge. It is a cauldron – whirlpools of grey and blue with a distinct battle line dividing these two great and terrible oceans, locked now in conflict. The gale snatches every word away; tears at our faces; it is unbelievably exhilarating. But when we turn to go back inside, the wind flattens me against the curve of the wall. I can barely move. He is ahead trying to force open the door in the teeth of something absolutely furious by now. I marvel how I am never afraid if he is there. He dispels my timidity. He finally manages to open the door, gashing his hand in the process, before he drags me through to safety. I am always surprised at how strong he is. He does not appear to be built strongly – but he is all steel. We are laughing now, inside the lighthouse. We wind our way down the stairs like naughty children and present ourselves to the alarmed attendant who reaches for the first-aid box and puts a No Entry sign on the door we have just emerged through – the last to climb the stairs that day.

... 'five or six weeks'.

I was becoming very familiar with Mount Wilga. I knew most of the recovering patients by sight. No matter what their physical handicaps, they all looked much stronger, robuster, than Eric. Some of them departed during our time there. Glance into a room, and the bed is empty, an over-zealous tidiness prevailing, a sudden drop in the temperature ... not for long – an ambulance arrives, or special taxi, and another guest at the health farm takes up residence.

Everyone, it seemed, recognized me, but I was treated with great tact, and our privacy was guaranteed by some sort of tacit understanding. This was much appreciated as it gave me an opportunity to wander at will, knowing that conversation need not necessarily have to be engaged in, and if it did, that it would never dwell on me or my long career. The only change to this guarded anonymity of mine happened one day when I found a bunch of flowers on one of Eric's tables. There was a card, which I prepared to read to him. But it was a card for me, anonymous, expressing sympathy and understanding, and contained the wish that one day I would be returning to the work that 'has given so many of us such pleasure over the years'. I was enormously touched by this gesture, and the giver's anonymity was strictly guarded by all, though there were many knowing smiles. All they would say was that the flowers had been handed over by a patient as she was leaving. I did notice that the room opening off Eric's shared bathroom was vacant for a day or two.

Eric would often be wheeled to the gazebo. It was a charming retreat, mostly in the sun, and he saw many of his visitors there. One lacked all sense of the purpose of Mount Wilga at such times. We could be serving tea after a tennis match – a deceptive ease and leisureliness pervading the afternoons. Eric's speech was still short of the desired, still filled with wonderful substitutions, but he maintained the social niceties with becoming ease. People gradually learned not to ask too many leading questions. Our then manager of the framing outlet at North Sydney, Lyn Haddrick, visited, and told him of the difficulty she was facing deciding what to do with her life. The framing shop was on the market and Lyn was quite unsure as to whether she should come to the Crows Nest shop or, indeed, move elsewhere. She had turned to Eric time and again for problem solving, and the habit was dying hard. He listened thoughtfully, nodding as the facts, the pros and cons, were presented. 'You've got some decisions to make, haven't you.' 'What are my options?' He leaned forward, and after a long pause for deliberation said, 'Well, Lyn . . . you can either do this – or you can do that.'

And Solomon, well pleased with himself, sank back into his throne. And winked.

Lyn thanked him and from that moment began the difficult journey of solving all problems by herself.

His room was always full of flowers. At that time of year the wattle was in bloom and we kept a bowl of it near the window. The Japanese maple, too, was afire and there would be a branch or two, making another glow. And pots of cyclamens, ferns, hothouse blooms. It took ten minutes or so, first thing every morning, to get through the gardening. But that room had the best of atmospheres, carrying right through to the garden outside. He could not have been in a better place and we were grateful that life, that Eric's 'tasks', proceeded as if his state were no different from that of all the other recovering patients. He was the ideal pupil, stretching himself still further in achievement. For a time we could all forget those haunting numbers, five or six ... feel we might make them, too, stretch ...

On the Saturday after the Queen's Birthday feast we brought him home again. Jonathan had returned to New Guinea, so it was Phillip who went to Mount Wilga on the Friday to master the intricacies of the journey; learn the extent to which Eric must, himself, be able to help.

This time, a more subdued meal. I cooked veal, cooked it slowly on the stove. It was to be tender as butter to aid his slight difficulty with swallowing.

This day the swallowing was markedly more difficult and there was one terrible moment when he choked badly and I thought, Oh, God, I've killed him, as we clustered about, waiting for the spasm to pass. But such a moment can colour an entire day. He did not seem as joyous as he had on that first great day, and was obviously tired. Anxieties flickered all round – but he was here, we could touch him, he existed, which can be the sum total of all one wants.

Fairly early into the afternoon he decided he should return. I went back with him this time, stayed awhile, saw him settled.

On the way out I spoke to Dawn, one of the senior sisters who was often on duty at night, found myself talking about the five or six weeks' prognosis.

'Ruth, I find I am never able to predict anything in these cases. It is *quite* impossible to say when someone will die.'

I thanked her. She was a quiet, reserved woman, who had been nursing for many years. I never doubted her deep wisdom and was grateful for it ... sensed I could be drawing on it ...

On the Sunday, in the afternoon, Eric was wheeled

to the gazebo. It was quite cold, but he was warmly dressed, blankets around him. He liked being outside. I had heard from our friend, Susan Bradley, with whom we had stayed in the Kimberley. She was passing through Sydney and said she would be visiting him. I asked him if she had called yet. He was disappointed that she had not. Another friend visited him, then a colleague from AWA days who had worked as second in command to Eric, years before. A lovely man. Eric was tiring, so they left, and then in the nick of time Susan appeared. Like the vodka on the flight home, she injected warmth and life into him, his face ironed out and he was right back in the world. Perhaps if we had suggested two weeks in the Kimberley he might have clawed back the months ...

It became quite cold, so I called a porter and we took him back into his room. He opted to go straight to bed, and soon I kissed him and said good-bye.

JUNE 15: I am having breakfast prior to going to Mount Wilga. Breakfasting alone; reading the paper; spreading the marmalade ...

Nothing unique about this. I have breakfasted alone these many years. He and I did not breakfast together – except when we were on holiday, and breakfast on holiday, by virtue of our otherwise solitary states during that first meal of the day, was an added fillip, a special treat, to be lingered over. We had breakfast together, too, when he visited me in other cities when I was on tour. In the daily business of living, however, Eric and I did not break bread together at the beginning of the day.

I remember we did not start out in this solitary fashion. When we were first married we lived in Wentworth Avenue in Vaucluse, on the ridge. We had an eccentric garden flat in the basement of a witch's house, complete with tower – and witch. The view was spectacular – we looked out onto the tops of oleanders and eucalypts that tumbled down the slope into Parsley Bay. Because of the vegetation we were not conscious of many other houses – although the odd red-tiled second storey could occasionally be glimpsed. For the rest, we were on the Riviera. A sensual, warm landscape for our sensual, warm days. We had friends over occasionally, we spoke to the witch and her ancient husband when this could not be avoided, but mostly we were, not surprisingly, entirely wrapped in one another. Our very first taste of cohabiting.

And we had breakfasts together. We passed the butter, we spread the marmalade, we drank – the tea for me, the coffee for him (sharing a pot of tea was something else that never occurred in our marriage) – we gazed at the view, the birds, one another. And then the terrible day, some weeks into our marriage, that Eric's eyes strayed to the paper at the side of his plate. I went into the radio studio that morning, and announced to all – and with a deep sense of personal loss – that the honeymoon was over. Eric was reading the paper at breakfast.

Admittedly, we still sat at the same table, sharing the news instead of gazing at one another – or rather *he* shared the news with *me,* I being relegated to a more inferior section of the paper, somewhere past page five.

What finally ended our breakfasts together, though, was his escaping early enough to miss the chaos of a *family* breakfast once the family, in the fullness of time, had reached a total of five. Breakfast during the childhood years passed, as in households the world over, minus the head of the household who has sensibly by that time realised his presence is required urgently elsewhere – or at the very least, that he needs to have his head stuck behind the pages of a newspaper to keep abreast.

When that sitcom childhood stage finally ended, I found I *preferred* breakfast on my own, thank you very much – and I wanted a whole newspaper to myself. Thus our solitary breakfasts became set in concrete.

Mind you, we always walked together before breakfast, travelling, for some reason, in the reverse direction to most of the other walkers, which was quite charming because it meant we greeted faces not backs and could say 'Good morning' brightly, many times. Even that early morning communion ended when the traffic became so impossible Eric decided to leave home at six. He then walked all round North Sydney, including the oval, and back to Crows Nest, where his day and his breakfast now started. He reported that the walkers around Crows Nest and

North Sydney were much less friendly – no one said 'Good morning' and he, too, gradually lost heart. Up to the time we left Sydney, Eric was walking two kilometres every working day – and on Sundays plunging into the bush at the bottom of the street with me. Sundays for pleasure, weekdays for health.

... and he might just as easily have spent that time sleeping, picking flowers, writing love letters ...

JUNE 15 is a Monday, and I am glancing at the television guide, deciding, while spreading the marmalade, what will be worth looking at this evening. Looking at television at night is one of the ordinary things I do in the midst of this extraordinary life I now lead.

Suddenly the phone breaks through. I answer it, a woman's voice says, 'It's Mount Wilga,' and I am on red alert even before she tells me that Eric has 'had a fainting spell in the shower and could I come please?' She gathers I am in pieces and adds 'No, don't worry, he's recovered, (What does that mean!?) but I think you should come.'

I am above the speed limit that morning on Pacific

Highway – it takes forever to break free of Hornsby, but eventually I am turning into Mount Wilga; I park; I race down the corridor; and at last I am in his room. It seems packed with people – nurses and both Dr Ragu and Dr Buckley at the bedside. They are speaking loudly and clearly to him – 'Eric, can you look directly at me. No, not just turn your head, can you turn your eyes to me?' It goes on for awhile, and they decide they will retreat, and just one nurse is left. I go to Eric. His eyes have swivelled around to the right side of his head, and he can only look towards the corner of his room near the door. So I go around to that side of the bed, where he will see me. 'Well! What have you been up to,' I say to him. He grins at me and a sort of a laugh comes out. 'Can't leave you for a minute, can I!' I stay with him for awhile, hating the look of him. His eyes seem to have lost their colour. They are muddy. I am able to leave him on the pretext of getting coffee, and swiftly join the two doctors, who are waiting for me.

It seems Eric, in all likelihood, has had either a blood clot to the brain, or the cancer has finally landed there. They will be sending him to The San tomorrow for a scan. The ambulance will be leaving as early as possible, but no one can be sure at just what time. He will be accompanied by a nurse and whoever else from the family wishes to go. 'Yes,' I say. Dependent upon the result, Eric may be re-admitted to The San – a prospect I cannot even allow myself to dwell on for an instant. He is happy and cared for where he is. He has had to make too many changes since that first admission in Venice those few short, unbelievably long months ago.

I make the necessary phone calls and Anna decides to catch the train to Sydney. She will stay the night with me. Jane will meet her at the station this afternoon, and I shall spend the day at the hospital.

I return to him.

He is reasonably comfortable, propped up, lying on his back, but still the eyes are twisted towards the corner of the room. He does not speak much, when he does his voice is much lighter in tone, although of course it is lighter in strength, too. Eric has – had – a fine speaking voice, deepish in register, light baritone, and he had a most pleasant singing voice, too, apart from the slight disadvantage of not being able to sing in tune. And as well as being lighter now, his voice has developed a slow country feel to it, very, very endearing ...

I sit with him all that day, except to replenish the coffee or tea. I feed him. He eats with enjoyment still, the last pleasure he will give up. Occasionally he says the odd word, but mostly we are peaceful. Once he says, very clearly, 'Mother' with his open eyes fixed on the corner near the door. Sometimes through that day he says 'Mum', once, 'Mummy'. I have the odd sensation that my late mother-in-law may slip through the door at any moment, laden with treats.

His pulse, as always, is strong. When Jonathan accompanied him for a special heart scan in Venice, there were many exclamations at the strength of it. Boom ... boom ... boom ...

Odd to remember that on the first day, the first momentous day, that he opened the door of the small framing outlet at Crows Nest – out on our own after nearly twenty years of corporate engineering life (more than thirty years for him if you add the years before we were married) – odd to remember, that on that first nervous day a relative, hitherto unknown, came to see him. The relative was in his thirties and had been stricken with very serious heart disease. So serious that he was urged to contact all his relatives to warn them of their highly vulnerable state. This information, coupled with the fact that Eric's father died at fifty, his maternal grandmother in her thirties, his uncle at an early age – all of coronary disease – left Eric with only one medical concern. Cholesterol was checked regularly, diet was watched -- and he walked, he walked ... My hand at his wrist attests to the success of this discipline – boom ... boom ... boom – thick and heavy. We might wish over the coming days – hours? – that he had not been so diligent ...

Jane arrives during the morning. Eric is disturbed to see her. She should be at work, therefore her presence indicates that this – incident – is serious. Among the staff there seems a sense of imminence ...

Eric is very quiet through most of this day, peaceful. He is not on any drugs other than his blood-controlling ones, and he has Normison at night if he is having trouble sleeping. Nothing else. He is never anxious or restless. Listening to the music, but no longer interested in Barry Humphries.

I am able to eat at Mount Wilga that day and on subsequent days all of us may. We are offered soup and rolls. Sometimes if all of us are there at the one time, this will be set up in the conference/ television room. Occasionally others will be in this room, but as often as not we are quite private.

Jane meets Anna in the late afternoon. Eventually, Anna and I have to say good-bye to him, but we assure him that we will be there early the next day for our ambulance ride. Jane stays with him.

JUNE 16: Anna and I arrive early. There are some unfamiliar faces among the nursing staff today. This is the time of year when some of the nurses are sitting for exams, so there are agency nurses filling the gaps. We meet the nurse who will accompany Eric to The San. She looks the epitome of efficiency – stoutly fitted out in navy blue uniform, badges.

Eric is resigned to the long day as he sets off . . .

In the midst of these journeys – and I think we all know now we are, inescapably, on the last, uncharted journey – in the midst of it all when you really ache to halt time, time sometimes will *be halted; but then you discover that is not what you want either. The day will be just a day wasted, or so it seems – a hiatus.*

Held up at a border crossing where the town has no character and there is no inducement to explore. You draw a line through the diary to show that nothing happened – or that you wish to obliterate what did happen.

We manage to find him! He is on the first floor in a curtained area. He is as comfortable as is possible in the circumstances, his stretcher facing the windows, curtains drawn back. People come and go along the corridor in front of him. He will be there for most of this day looking out the window because, although the procedure itself takes only a short time, we will have to wait on the availability of an ambulance for his return journey – praying there will be no requirement for him to remain at The San.

We take it in turns to rub his chest, hold the cup and straw to his lips, feed him. We hurry to the café when he goes off for the scans; we hurry back. Then we take it in turns to escape for awhile. He becomes very cold, so Anna tries to warm him – rubs his chest. While she is massaging, he looks towards the windows and says very clearly, 'I can see her. She's waiting for me. But I'm not ready yet.'

Later, Anna asks, 'Do you want anything, Dad?'

Bleakly, from him, 'I'm just hoping for a bit of luck.'

As are we all …

The day winds on, and by mid-afternoon we have an ambulance. The results are available, but not proffered. We are advised that Dr Ragu will be notified immediately and if we are impatient for information we should phone him. Anna, who is about to catch a train home, is indeed impatient, so I phone Dr Ragu as Anna heads the car towards Wahroonga Station. We learn that there is bleeding in the brain, which probably – certainly? – means that the cancer has migrated to another site. Armed with this information, Anna will make plans to return to Sydney on Thursday and then stay with me.

JUNE 17: Jane and I meet Stephen Buckley. No medical procedures are contemplated at The San. Stephen accepts that it is cancer in the brain – there is bleeding occurring; we are quite possibly down to 'hours . . .'

I think it has all happened so quickly, leaped upon us while we were looking the other way . . .

Eric will now require palliative care. Mount Wilga is a rehabilitation hospital. There is a specialist palliative care hospital at Wahroonga, to which Eric would, in the normal course of events be conveyed. I dread the next inevitable sentence – and, when it comes, am unable to believe the words that I do hear –

'He can stay here, you know. We can look after him.'

It takes awhile before the full implications sink in. When they do, my gratitude and relief are without constraint . . . looking back, I can say that those words were, quite simply, the loveliest I had heard over our entire adventure. What they meant, of course, was that the roller coaster had finally come to a halt – and at the most harmonious of stations . . .

At the time, I am only conscious of a huge weight being lifted. Eric can stay where he is ... no more packing, no more transfers, no new environment, no new faces – why, we are so happy, we are skipping around a maypole he and I ...

... he can stay ... he can stay ... round and round – then skip away ...

... festooned and garlanded ...

On the medical side, we are advised that he will go on steroids for a few days. This will reduce the swelling in the brain – will also, we are told, induce a feeling of euphoria. This will only be temporary because the treatment will not continue past three or four days. (I think three days of euphoria are not to be sneezed at.) I thank Stephen Buckley. I wonder if he knows what a great present he has given us!

Sitting with Eric later, I look around the room. His final abode is very comfortable now. Perhaps this is one of my better talents. I can always make the dwelling of the moment serene – even during the shortest of stays.

I want this for myself always, but even more have I wanted it for him, for whom conflict, discord – particularly over the last few years – have become untenable. Whatever other lamentable falls from grace there have been, a capacity to create our own 'serene state' I have managed. No wonder we headed for Venice – seduced as we were by a name ...

The Serene City, of course, had revealed herself, at times, as anything but – becoming cross-hatched with discord and unpredictability. On the other hand, by virtue of her very unpredictability, we had at least had the advantage of a most valuable, if swift, apprenticeship.

Occasionally, very softly from him, 'Mummy ...'

We are still deeply connected, not even needing to talk. After a time I ask, 'Would you like some music?' The soft country drawl comes back, 'If you like.' I move to the CD player as he continues, '*I* can't stand it! You can have it, though!' My hand withdraws and I return to my chair, grinning at him, his eyes glinting back. They seem to be a little better, not so muddy, not twisted. Perhaps the steroid is beginning to work.

The nurses come and go, the drinks come and go. One, a highly nutritious glug that packs a punch. He has special jugs of this concoction in the fridge. 'Mr Phillips', they say. I help feed him. No pretence at his feeding himself now. There will be no more visits to the dining room, but he will move to the chair in his room occasionally, and a wheelchair is always there for his use. Our daughters come and go – very few other visitors now. It will be just family and the closest.

Jonathan has already spoken from New Guinea to Stephen Buckley, and the advice is that Jonathan return. He will be arriving late Thursday, but we don't tell Eric yet.

JUNE 18: Dr Ragu wants to speak to us, so Anna, Jane and I join him in his office. He proposes, for our consideration, the cessation of the anti-clotting drugs. I am appalled. We sit there, trying to summon up arguments against the suggestion. The decision has to be ours – or mine, really, I suppose. It is inescapable. It is a truly awful moment. It is too – precipitate ... I need to sit by a river for awhile ...

Then, from Dr Ragu, very quietly, 'What are we trying to do here! We have lost the battle.'

Trudging through the snow from Moscow, lines and lines of the defeated.

'All right. Yes,' I hear myself say.

No flag at half mast? No Last Post?

'It is the right decision.'

Is it? So simply taken. This unwinding of his life I am not prepared for.

That afternoon Petrea King comes to see him. I had asked him if he would like to see her and he had said he would. I knew how special she was, but I was not sure how he might react to her.

I had met Petrea some years before after a performance of *Lost In Yonkers,* the Neil Simon play that began its touring season at the Theatre Royal in Sydney. Often a charitable group will take part of the house to raise funds, and there is always a function afterwards to which the cast and crew are invited. I seldom go to these occasions, mostly because I am too tired. But this night, for some reason, I found myself attending. The charity was Petrea's Quest for Life Foundation. This Foundation aids and encourages all who are threatened with serious illness. (I am unable to use the word 'terminal' – it is not in Petrea's vocabulary except as a place for buses at the end of the day.) She and those who work for her are able to enrich life for as long as life lasts. Her Foundation also cares for and supports the carers of such people. The evening was such a delightful one, and I met so many positive and attractive people, that I began an association with Petrea, which has enabled me at times to support her. Many of the people at that after-theatre party had lost loved ones, but were still active in supporting her fund raising. Petrea herself has experienced the very situations that she now assists others through – her 'terminal' condition having vanished some years ago. Petrea's work is an adjunct to medical procedures and treatments. She is, quite simply, one of life's most gifted and generous.

Petrea had visited me early on our return from

Venice. We talked for an hour or more, and her practical and intelligent advice on how to preserve myself during this 'process' had proved invaluable.

Petrea arrives, armed with some meditation tapes. I tell her what he has said about listening to music, so they are not proffered during her time with him. She talks easily, not about anything specifically, but every so often you can see how skilfully she is assessing him. She asks if he would like a gentle massage, which on his assent, she starts. She suggests that massaging the feet is especially helpful, and in a second is smoothly proceeding – still talking quietly, perceptively – with a massage I am unconsciously absorbing. I cannot remember a word she said to him, but I remember with clarity the atmosphere she created. Walking to her car she says, 'You don't have to worry. He's in good shape.' I am left with the impression that Eric is graduating summa cum laude and am conscious of a thrill of pride.

Later in the afternoon, my nephew, David, and his wife, Susan, come to see him; Helen and Bruce, Anna's inlaws; Kirrily – everyone saddened, everyone still in a state of disbelief. Jonathan arrives at night from New Guinea.

JUNE 19: Jonathan goes in to him for the first time. His father cries deeply. 'I know why you're here,' and for the first time he knows death in his gut. Then, as with everything else, accepts. We are in and out, we take it in turns, or we all gather about him. We protect him, we cherish him. He is surrounded.

... and we were comforted in our sadness by his complete lack of fear, his acceptance and his love for us. We are lucky ...

Lisa is sketching him. She cannot think of anything else to do. She focuses on the pencil strokes, frowning with concentration. I wonder what the result will be.

Paula Peres drops in to see him. He can still sparkle at her presence. They joke a bit. She sits for a time; massages him. She had made him very fit. Fit for a marathon.

After our soup and rolls, I go home for awhile. Anna is there. I go first to the letterbox, pull out two letters in the same hand – a hand I recognize. One is addressed to him, one to me. I tear into them. They are from his sister.

Almost fourteen years earlier there had been a rift between this brother and sister, the details of which no longer matter. It was a rift from which Eric did not really recover. I do not think he believed it could have happened. Once or twice over the intervening years he had endeavoured to resolve the situation, but had finally accepted that this was not going to happen. He seldom referred to it, but part of him from that time was in shadow. There was a corner the light did not reach. And while it was scarcely at the forefront of his thoughts, it was undeniably *there.* A death in the family, but without possibility of easing the grieving.

I had not been in touch with her, but I knew she would be aware of Eric's state. Sometimes, as his situation became more dire, I came very close to asking for a rapprochement, but instinctively knew that, even if this were responded to, it would not work. It had to be her decision, her desire. It was at the second level of my consciousness from the moment I knew he was not going to survive. And now, here it was. Just sitting quietly in the letterbox. Unforced. I read both letters, folded mine away, raced back to Mount Wilga with Anna. We had to hurry ... I walked into his room; no great change, thank God; as we had left him. I requested that everyone leave us and sat down to read, which was terribly difficult, because not only was he crying, but it was almost impossible for me to get the words out. What a joyful sound was there! 'Thank her! Thank her!' he cried, over and over. 'Tell her I love her. Thank her. Do thank her!'

You could say in the nick of time.

I was alone with him for awhile after struggling through her letter – trying to get myself under some sort of control. He had received the perfect gift – and one that finally released him.

In that sense, you could also say, a happy ending ...

JUNE 20: He has everyone in his room today at different times. All the grandchildren, John and Phillip. Everyone saying good-bye without saying good-bye.

Later, he is restless and not very comfortable. Irritable, too, though not ever, in these last days, with me. Kirrily is with Jane as they try to make him comfortable. The setting of the back rest on the bed will not satisfy him – up and down they go, trying every ratchet. 'No! No!' he groans. He can't get comfortable. They work frantically, but nothing appeases and finally, 'You're both bloody useless,' he tells them. They manage to soothe him, finally.

Kirrily leaves. 'I can't believe I won't be seeing him again.'

Later – it is sunny and pleasant, and he is more cheerful – Anna and Jane have him transferred to his wheelchair and they take him for a walk, round and round the garden …

… He was impatient to go outside, bored with being in his room, bored with the whole process of dying. 'Let's go now,' *he said. 'I can't wait,' and moving the wheelchair with his good leg he laughed,* 'This *is* fun.'

As he was wheeled through the garden he kept saying, 'This is beautiful. It's so *beautiful.' And we could see it, too. Each leaf was more leaflike, each flower more like a flower. In those last days his desire to live every moment, to make it count, was inspiring and infectious.*

And we were comforted in our sadness by his complete lack of fear, his acceptance and his love for us ...

JUNE 21: It has become quite cold. The euphoria from the steroids has certainly passed. He is uncomfortable and tired of it all. His son-in-law, John, does say good-bye. 'Have fun!' is his response. Anna will stay on with me.

In the afternoon, he asks what the time is. 'Only four o'clock! This seems to be taking forever!' he groans. Jonathan lifts him out of bed into the wheelchair and he and Lisa take him out, shrouded in blankets for a race all around the garden and the old house next door. I watch out the window. It is grey, grey ... He is crouched low in the wheelchair, a blanket over his head. He seems tiny. They come back and his spirits have lifted. He simply cannot get comfortable now. It is probably the condition of his bones.

I, too, wonder how long this will take.

The staff are wonderful to him. Maureen, who is

often on at night, sits with him and holds his hand if he cannot sleep.

There are a lot of us making this journey. We keep one another going. We seem quite cheerful at times. Just at times ...

JUNE 22: He is asked if he would like morphine and says, 'Yes.' He begins with two and a half millilitres. Fairly light. He is mostly having just liquid now. The thickish mixture can be fed to him with a spoon. One or all the family are here throughout the day. We leave at night reluctantly, but with relief. Sometimes two of us will speed off during the day for a cup of good coffee and a view of the world. We touch him a lot, gently rub his chest, take his hand. He is more comfortable since the morphine, and not so befuddled as to be unaware. He is waiting, we are waiting, we are doing it together.

We have had to think about a funeral. Certain procedures are relentless. One has to think ahead, while at the same time only wanting to be entirely immersed in the moment.

I felt sure in my mind what I wanted for the funeral. I needed only to talk to him about it. So I did. And he wept. But was happy with what I was sure was right for us. A funeral in the church we had been married in. The church his parents had been married in. We both wanted our friend Howard Hollis, now retired to Melbourne, to participate.

So we set the plans in motion.

I do not believe this is happening . . .

The room itself remains an enjoyable place to be. The sun floods in at certain times of the day. The staff come in and pamper and spoil, and he is still able to lap that up with great enjoyment. He has, over these weeks, months, been disagreeable sometimes, occasionally demanding, impatient, but not once – ever – from him, the slightest vestige of self-pity or anger. I am not sure how usual this is.

Once, Anna said to him, 'Oh, Dad! I'm so sorry

you're so sick!' He smiled and shrugged. 'That's life!' he said, and got on with the business of dying.

JUNE 23: We are told that in the early hours of the morning, Eric consumed a large bowl of jelly! Everyone most surprised.

Today a social worker says she is worried about me, and him. Shouldn't he be transferred to the Palliative Care Hospital? 'No!' I reply shortly. Later, Stephen Buckley tells me of his qualifications in this area, and those of some of the staff. I do not need any convincing.

Once, Eric opens his eyes, looks at me and says, quite sternly, 'Now *you've* got to be tough.' I smile at him. 'Don't worry.'

Each day he is closer, but no way of knowing how close. The strain is beginning to tell. There has never been any other life. There will never be any other life.

But we have one final decision to take. Drs Buckley and Ragu need to know our feelings about administering liquid intravenously. It may prolong his life. It will help prevent dehydration. Do they proceed with it? This is the hardest of the decisions – and, as always, it has to be ours. Jonathan finds it particularly hard. I think he feels it is unthinkable to deny him – what? – comfort? Finally, it comes down to me. I do not know. How can I?

Then Dr Ragu says very quietly, 'He's in God's hands now. It doesn't matter whether you're a Hindu or what you are. I can tell you, he's in God's hands.'

So I say, 'All right.'

And anyway, I discover there are other ways to get liquid into him.

JUNE 24: His morphine dose has been increased to five millilitres. He is weaker each day, but only minimally. The Reverend Richard Hurford, the Rector of St James', visits him. Richard asks him if he would like to be anointed. Eric says, 'Yes.' Does he mind? Does he not? Is he indifferent? No way of knowing. But the four of us gather around the bed, and Richard explains each step, how he is anointing him with oil blessed last Easter by the bishop. It is all very simple and quick.

And then our priest departs ...

JUNE 25: One of the nurses drags on a pair of surgical gloves. She wraps some gauze around her forefinger, drenches it in water, and holds it to his lips. He sucks greedily, and, it seems, enjoyably. She tells me I can do this. So I draw on surgical gloves, wrap gauze around my finger and hold it to his lips. It is like feeding a baby kangaroo. He sucks greedily, and I repeat and repeat. I think this is a much more personal way of delivering water. It is not much more than water from here on. Later in the afternoon, one of the older sisters appears. She wipes out his mouth for him, sponges inside his mouth for him. She has not bothered to pull on any surgical gloves and I think, Why in God's name am I putting on gloves for my husband! I feel ashamed. And from that moment the sucking roo has a more satisfying pull on the teat. Our tiny, sensual moment …

He is propped up all the time. Nurses come and go, sponging, trying not to disturb, succeeding in making his life comfortable, cherished.

I am the main one in his sights now. He is focused on me, so that it becomes difficult to go away from him. He sleeps a little. I am conscious of great weariness every time I leave the room. The others, Anna, Jane, Jonathan, Lisa, alternate between the bedside and the conference room, which we seem to have taken over for much of the day. Sometimes, a blessed walk down along the high ridge of the road. We walk quickly, bush all around us and sometimes take in the garden of the old house on the way back. It is really winter.

JUNE 26: There seems little change. His eyes still riveted on me when I am there. We keep the liquids up. He is made comfortable – they make sure he is turned regularly. In the afternoon I am trudging along the corridor, and Paula Peres approaches. She is concerned for me, wondering how long I can keep this up. It had occurred to me.

'Would it be better if you had him at home? You'd rest more.'

I am shaken and unsure what is best for either of us. I see Dawn later. Say to her, lightly, 'Will I still be coming here like this next Christmas?' She senses my need, my – almost – despair. There is a pause and then she says simply and deliberately, 'It won't be more than forty-eight hours now.' I believe her.

In the midst of all this grieving, but not yet grieving, the business of dying has to be coped with. We have to organize a funeral director, having no experience of these matters. We make our choice.

There is now someone else who is waiting ...

His breathing has become very strained, and it is not easy to be with him because it is distressing, but you have to be with him because he knows – is aware. I am in no doubt as to that.

It is very strange. In this busy environment, where so many are being readied for a return to life, here in the very middle is a beautiful space where someone is being readied, guided, led by the hand, to death.

We have arrived at the week-end. The week-end of the forty-eight hours. On the Saturday, he is still aware of me, knows I am there, but on the Sunday, it seems he no longer does and I am desolate. I feel there is no more connection between us, that perhaps, for me, he is already dead. I am completely empty. Barren.

The forty-eight hours pass.

JUNE 29: This morning he is propped up, and he is on his back. I am standing at the foot of his bed. I am alone with him. His eyes are open and he is holding my gaze with the greatest intensity I have experienced in our whole, nearly forty-one, years. As surely as when he shouted with joy in San Giovanni e Paolo that first time in Intensive Care, 'I KNOW *YOU*!' does he know me now!

His eyes are so blue. I say to him, 'Have you stolen the colour from my eyes?' I find, without knowing it, that I am massaging his feet, just the way I had seen Petrea do it. His eyes do not leave me, and I begin to sing to him, as I did on that first terrible night in Venice. But this time I go on and on, waiting for the eyes to release me. I sing every song that comes into my head, massaging, massaging. I sing every verse of *Waltzing Matilda* as taught to me by Auntie Ethel when I was a little girl. I sing and I sing ... and he finally closes his eyes. For those minutes – hours? – how many I have no idea, time had become meaningless.

In our isolated cocoon, he and I tunnelled into one another.

On this Monday evening, Jane, Anna and I left Mount Wilga at around six o'clock. Jonathan and Lisa maintained the watch. Anna's daughters, Madeleine and Celeste, were waiting for us. Jane returned to her home, and Anna and I stayed with the granddaughters, preparing dinner.

Jonathan rang to say there had been a change, a profound change to his father's eyes.

I telephoned Dawn; asked her should we return. The slightest pause, and then, 'Yes.'

I phoned a neighbour and she came to the house to be with the two children. The older one, Madeleine, was upset, wanting to come with us, but we persuaded her that this would not be the right thing. The change in his appearance over the past week since she had last seen him had been dramatic and painful.

My neighbour arrived, and Anna waited for Jane, who was on her way. Madeleine was still upset, so I took an old copy of *The Ancient Mariner* from the bookshelves. It has beautiful illustrations, and it seemed the best thing in the world to be looking at, dipping into, at this moment . . .

> O sleep! it is a gentle thing,
> Beloved from pole to pole!
> To Mary Queen the praise be given!
> She sent the gentle sleep from Heaven,
> That slid into my soul . . .

. . . and my neighbour began reading it to her as I left.

All who are living at Mount Wilga, temporarily, are sleeping, resting, when I arrive. It is very quiet, wonderfully peaceful, lights dim. I hurry to his room. Jonathan vacates the chair and I sit by my husband's side. I do not like this at all. His breathing is desperately laboured. He lies on his side, eyes closed, beyond (*or is he?*) all human contact. Jonathan takes up a position on the other side of the bed, diagonally opposite. I am conscious of the precision of the lines, as if drawn, between us. Jonathan, his father's head on the pillow, me. A precise, narrow triangle. To the right of Jonathan I notice the clock with its large numbers that Jonathan had bought at K Mart – an easy clock for his father to read. It reads 9.20.

I sit there for a moment. Jonathan speaks sternly, 'Take his hand!'

I do not want to, but do. My hand slips under the covers, finds a kangaroo paw. It is warm.

The terrible breathing continues.

We remain like this. Jonathan is immovable. Again, time has lost itself.

My eyes do not leave Eric's face, but I have no confidence that I matter to him now.

He seems quite alone.

The breathing continues ... each breath a mighty struggle ...

... but each breath keeps coming ...

The world is waiting. The world has reduced itself to this triangle of soft light in a familiar room.

We wait, and we wait. I cannot believe the breathing. It seems so – courageous, strong. I feel his strength could carry him to the end of time, the three of us there in our capsule, spinning away – maintained only by his great strength, his command ...

so much strength, so much will, from this pitifully reduced being …

Still, the triangle holds. Nothing moves – only the chest on the bed.

… two sounds … a ticking clock and the awful breathing …

… then, as I watch, there is a mighty intake of breath, reaching way, way out – he is gulping in the universe …

… then, silence. My husband has stopped breathing.

I am not sure what should be happening now … what is the … form?

My voice – I think it is my voice, 'Shouldn't we call someone?'

Jonathan is rooted to his point of the triangle.

'Ring the bell!' he orders. 'It's near you!'

… so I do.

I am conscious of a change to the kangaroo paw. It is gradually getting colder.

Fiona is at the bedside in a second, a stethoscope held to his throat.

'Is he dead?' I hear myself say.

'If he isn't,' she says very softly, 'it will be any minute.'

There is no sound from him. There has been no sound since that last mighty gulp.

At that moment his daughters fly into the room.

'Come quickly! Come quickly!' says Fiona, leaving his side.

They stand by him, and after a moment, he lets out a deep, soft sigh.

And then, he does die.

My eyes go straight to the clock. It reads 9.40.

How to describe this? No way at all.

I remember sinking back into my chair and I know I am smiling and that, mixed with everything else, there is such a happiness, but no, happiness is not my state – such a state, then, as I have not before experienced. The four of us are alone; he has no more struggling to do; it is wonderful for him. I am smiling for, and *at,* him – not at the figure in the bed, necessarily, but at him, there, *everywhere* within this blessed space. Blessed, because indisputably he is sharing the moment with us. No question. No question. It is the most precious moment I have known; it is the most *surprising* moment because entirely unexpected. And if this moment I can keep, then nothing more do I need, now or ever. We are not, you see, and this you must believe, in an empty room; but in a space suffused. We are – golden; we seem for a tiny fragment of time, holy; a medieval painting. If only we could be captured as we are now we would be free forever (with our secret), untrammelled ...

... only hang on to it ... oh! only hang on to it ...

... I do not want to go ...

But, inevitably, we are led from our space, and already it begins to fade ...

What we are left with, before grief takes over, is, first and foremost, I suppose, the most immense sense of relief. So much of these last weeks has seemed interminable, unable in any way to be ended; a continuum of new and unwillingly acquired knowledge – unlooked for knowledge. Precious knowledge. Will this knowledge fade, as the fairies faded from our childhood? Now that we have looked into the heart of things, will we *remain* ... unique ... or is the point of it all the actual *ordinariness* of the revelation? Always at hand, just waiting to be invited in ...

... oh, such an extraordinary, ordinary, time we have shared ...

We are ushered back into the combined television/ conference room where Lisa has been waiting out the night. She had foraged for some take-away, but I am not sure that we ate. Perhaps we did. Eventually, Stephen Buckley arrived. There is the business to be attended to. There is the business of the death certificate; there is the business of the funeral director; it all proceeds in the manner of these things, efficiently, coolly.

When it comes to the death certificate, I ask, with a degree of flippancy that is possibly faintly shocking, 'Well! What will *you* be putting on *this* death certificate, Stephen? Do we go for lung cancer or an aberrant blood clot?' 'Oh, lung cancer, of course,' says Stephen. 'The cause of death was lung cancer!'

In the event, the death certificate has a bit each way – every way –

CAUSE OF DEATH:

(I) a) Cerebral oedema 14 days
b) Metastatic lung cancer (brain secondaries) 28 days
c) Squamous cell or undifferentiated large cell carcinoma 3 months

(II) Antiphospholipid syndrome 3 months

Such a deal of complexity over such a short time.

We are all ushered back into his room. Fiona and her assistant have worked with tenderness and perception. He is now on his back, a rolled hand towel at his neck holding his head in place. On either side of his head, on the pillow, are the last two, tiny burnished leaves from the Japanese maple. On the bedside table, a Bible has been opened at Psalm 23. It is all done with the utmost thought. It does not really matter. The room is empty – even seems to have a different lighting state – brighter, flatter. The flowers, the pots, the cards, the artwork – all are still there, but this room is now foreign. We do not belong.

The journey has been completed, our companion escorted carefully to the border. He has gone. We are left.

A very terrible finality here in this room now. I cannot wait to leave.

There are tasks within the room still, of course. But one or other of the children will be attending to that. Drawers to be emptied, cupboard to be cleared, pots, artwork, messages, collected.

As for us – he and I have checked out of a room for the last time. We shall not be doing it again. Ever.

Before I leave, Jane, who has some instinct for these things, says, 'Look!' She is reading the psalm, but it is not the 23rd, it is the preceding psalm.

She hands it to me and I read,

'My heart has turned to wax and is melting ...'

I turn and walk out of Mount Wilga for the last time.

I do not have too clear a memory of the next few days. I think I slept through most of Tuesday. I remember the business of choosing a coffin, checking all the arrangements for the following Friday. I remember speaking to the director of music at St James', David Drew, persuading him, much to his surprise, to include a few bars of a twenties ballad in his beautiful opening processional music. I remember the rector visiting us and finalising all our choices for music and words. I remember the constant procession of flowers …

But I remember all this through a mist. I was on the far side of the mist. A shade. Insubstantial …

… my heart, you see, had turned to wax and was melting …

EPILOGUE

. . . Now I want
Spirits to enforce, art to enchant;
And my ending is despair
Unless I be relieved by prayer . . .

The Tempest
William Shakespeare

When I look back over the events I have been describing, I find there are many questions for which there will not be firm answers. I could ask, for instance, what it would have been like if we had not suddenly switched plans and gone to Venice instead of New York – or just about anywhere else in the world.

Venice seems a thoroughly modern city, with everything available at the push of a room-service bell; all difficulties able to be sorted out by a quick visit to a bank or a tourist office. Just change your money and make your purchases. And when you are going, the water taxi will be ready and waiting and you will leave Venice with a lump in your throat because you will never have seen anything more beautiful in your life.

The tourist, the traveller, reigns supreme, and the city bends in all directions to secure favours, assure contentment. But when you stop being a traveller, the masks are cast aside and you are staring at the true face of Venice. Unadorned, no paint, no silk and lustre to captivate, just the hardness and the toughness of Venetian reality. And you are forced to discover a matching toughness within yourself or you will sink like a pebble tossed into a fountain.

You must become the Venetian who does battle with the difficulties of the city on a daily basis. I speak here, of course, of the ordinary Venetian and not the beautiful birds of paradise who inhabit the grand palazzos and have as much to do with those who inhabit a few rooms as the high apartment dwellers of New York have to do with those who inhabit the streets.

I became that tougher Venetian, and, yes, if I had my wish, Eric's calamity would have happened anywhere but that city – a city that persuades you it knows all about the twentieth century, dwells easily within it. But cross that line from tourist to inhabitant, and Venice will bring you face to face with her other side; her medieval reality. A reality that, if peered into earlier from the comfort of leafy Sydney, might have curdled the blood.

Yet Venice gave me something else, something priceless that I cannot disown nor will ever now be without. Lodged within my soul are the miracles of Venice. I do not know how else to describe the highly unlikely, the against-all-odds events that happened there. The Serene City that keeps the secret of her serenity, perhaps, solely for those in deep need – and who will only be able to recognize it much later, in recollection.

At the beginning of these unusual events stands the stark fact, unknown by me till much later, that though Eric's dangerous blood condition by the time he reached hospital resided in its inability to coagulate, this bleeding would have been preceded by clotting within the blood vessels. In other words, for the first week of our 'holiday', Eric was producing clots that could have caused him, at any moment, to drop dead at my feet. That he did not is not by definition a miracle; it is just another strand in this devastating sequence of events.

In my dictionary, 'miracle' is described as – 'I. An extraordinary event attributed to some supernatural agency. II. Any remarkable occurrence ...' What he and I experienced in the real Venice were indeed extraordinary events, remarkable occurrences. Whether attributable to 'some supernatural agency' is not for me to say or to attempt to convince, it is simply for me to have experienced.

The first miracle, I believe, occurred in Venice on that Tuesday night in Intensive Care. Admitted by a specialist who was convinced that Eric was dying, he was resuscitated. The records show this. I think, without any doubt in my mind, that Eric should have died that night, every indication pointed to imminent death, and yet he came back. *Resuscitated,* one way or another. I do not attempt to interpret what his first words to me in Intensive Care meant. I only know that he said them. In Sydney, our surgeon friend, John Rogers, was convinced Eric was dying, that he would be dead before Anna arrived in Venice. And yet Eric did not die. He was alive against *all* the odds. A most remarkable occurrence.

The second miracle, by any definition, was the

fact of his escape from Venice. Everything was stacked against us, but somehow, yes, miraculously, at the last minute, even past the last minute when he had collapsed in the hospital, *this* most remarkable of occurrences proceeded. As it unfolded, it contained within it the miracle of his survival of the plane trip – again, *against all the odds.* He was either blessed with the most extraordinary will power, a power of mind that was pushing all the limits, or he was kept alive for some other reason.

The third miracle was the arrival of his sister's letter – the most important of the 'miracles' for Eric, the one that the others, perhaps, were moving towards; the one that allowed him, from the moment of my reading it to him, to leave us. Which he did.

I do not even touch on the extraordinary things he said occasionally. They were not drug induced because he was not on hallucinatory or narcotic drugs at the time. I must also point out that Eric himself had never shown any inclination towards supernatural or 'psychic' persuasions in his life. His discipline was science, and he was of the opinion that most mysteries had a simple answer. Which made it all the more extraordinary when he spoke, so naturally, in different terms from any he had ever used before.

I am happy with the possibility of 'miracles'. They do not perturb me. But I do not dwell on them. It just did not surprise me to learn that my Venetian Madonna was known as the Madonna of Victory ...

Whatever these musings, whatever the causes, these victories were hard won. They were also, for me, life changing. Over the months, particularly over the last weeks, I came to see with absolute clarity a side of Eric that had only been glimpsed previously. I do not wish to portray him as a saint. Eric was anything but that. He was difficult at times, unreasonable frequently, nit-picking and infuriating. I had never doubted, though, that he was *essentially* a good man. A creative man. An evolved man. I should know. I was the lucky recipient of his fine intelligence, his generosity and his utterly non-judgemental view of humankind.

But the closer he got to – the end? – the closer he seemed to be to this essence. In the grace of his dying, what I was looking at in its purest and simplest form was, I believe, goodness, the spirit ...

and – most miraculous of all – the inter-connectedness of this spirit. It joined the two of us and it fanned out … everything seemed connected at that most mysterious and wonderful of moments … that most revelatory of moments …

And that is what journeying to Venice and beyond was about.

Now my charms are all o'erthrown,
And what strength I have's mine own . . .

The Tempest
William Shakespeare

On the anniversary of Eric's death the family gathered at St James' for a private service. We were interring his ashes in the crypt of the church. This was the children's decision as much as mine. The ashes held little meaning for me. I would have been just as happy scattering them through the bush at the bottom of the street – or emptying them in the compost.

The ashes had been retrieved from the crematorium a month or two after his death. Jonathan had collected them in their large plastic container. I imagine an urn would present a greater aura of solemnity, bring a degree of dignity, make one take the contents more seriously, but this plastic container always seemed to me like something that should be going on a picnic.

After collecting the container, Jonathan placed it

on the passenger seat of his car, duly belted, and, as it was peak hour, took the liberty of travelling in the restricted transit lane, figuring that if stopped by the police they would have some difficulty arguing that he did *not* have a passenger.

While we were still undecided as to their ultimate resting place, the ashes stayed happily under a terracotta chimney pot in the back garden – right in the middle of the azaleas. If I sat on the back verandah, which I often do at dusk, I could keep an eye on him, settled there in a froth of blazing white as spring skipped through its paces.

Then, one day, early into the new year, after canvassing other prospects, we made the decision that if he was not going in the bush, he would be placed in a niche in the small columbarium at St James'.

One in all in, I thought, and decided to reserve a niche right next door for me. Everyone seemed relieved and satisfied.

Unfortunately, there had been a booking for a corporate luncheon at the crypt on our day. Ours was definitely not a movable feast, so we trusted to luck that all in our tiny band would be punctual.

Otherwise there was the prospect of the moment being intruded upon by happy laughter, loud voices, and the clinking of glasses.

Jonathan and Lisa were to travel with me, so they came to the house. We retrieved the ashes, and I suggested that Jonathan make an inspection just in case the odd snail had breached the defences. Just a spider's web he reported. 'Come and look.' I did not want to look, but did, to please him. Peering into the container at something that could have been a mix of chicken feed and rolled oats I thought, Well! How ridiculous! This is as much my man as the dynamic lifter.

Just the same, if I am honest, a strange sensation . . . Oh, yes.

Alas, poor Eric . . .

Deciding in what discreet covering to transport him caused a degree of to-ing and fro-ing, Jonathan refusing to carry him in a David Jones shopping bag. A suitcase seemed a little sinister, and an attaché case decidedly pompous. We finally settled for an anonymous and suitably sturdy plastic bag, and set forth.

We dropped Lisa at the church and proceeded to the carpark at the back of Sydney Hospital. Jonathan carried his father to the lift. We crowded in with two others, who smiled delightedly.

Shoulder to shoulder, waiting forever for the doors to close . . . the lift to ascend . . .

There is nothing quite like sharing a lift with people who do not know what you are carrying, when what you are carrying is a bag of someone's ashes. Nervous glances flick around the confined space from the guilty ones and it is not long before you feel the plastic bag has fluorescent tape all over it screaming *Dad's ashes! Dad's ashes!* When the doors finally opened, we bolted with all the speed of a brace of criminals.

Even walking down the street presented difficulties. The fear that a bicycle would bump into us, causing ashes to be scattered far and wide . . . or, worse, that we might be mugged.

At last we arrived at the church, where the secretary was waiting to open the crypt door. Her eyes travelled to the plastic bag, and we smiled nervously again. Fortunately, our rector, Richard, then arrived and he, of course, has no problem at all with ashes – no matter what the wrapping.

While waiting for Anna's family to appear I sat in the side chapel and gathered my thoughts. Unsure how I would react as the morning progressed, I was quite calm in the chapel. Jane, Phillip, and their children, Rebecca and Isobel, were quietly wandering about, looking at the memorial tablets, when the travellers arrived. We all grouped in the porch. Richard could not get over how much Anna's sons had grown in a year. 'You two must have been standing in fertiliser!' he exclaimed. There was nervous shuffling from the boys, a furtive inspection of footwear ...

Then, in a little while, we found ourselves in the tiny columbarium, lined with its niches. There was an altar, and we noted with pleasure that the flower arrangers had placed a beautiful vase on a pedestal for us. The door to one niche was open; we were shown the brief inscription on the brass plate that would be affixed later, and the short, simple service began. Grandson Ali handed over an origami bird fashioned by Madeleine, and this went into the niche with Eric's ashes. Richard told the children that they could come into this place whenever they wished, and that it would be a nice thing to just sit there and remember everything that their grandfather had done for them, and all that he meant to them.

Celeste was becoming a little voluble at this stage, and her Uncle Phillip picked her up. It was only then I noticed she was not wearing any panties; I hoped Richard was not going to be too bothered by the intrusion of a cherubic bottom into proceedings. As Celeste seemed to have been lifted straight off a Tiepolo ceiling, the bottom was not altogether inappropriate. My only worry was where she may have left her panties, and hoped it was not under one of the pews upstairs.

The caterers for the corporate luncheon had been extremely considerate, whispering instructions to one another as they set out plates and knives and forks, *very* quietly. As we left, the jovial corporate people were just gathering. The timing had worked splendidly.

Richard now steered us towards the children's chapel, the secret treasure in the crypt, with its fresco by the Turramurra artists – a group organized by the art critic and patron Ethel Anderson. Executed in the thirties, it is a delight of children, parents, frolicking – joyful happiness on all sides, with an unfinished span of the Harbour Bridge placing it precisely in time. Grace Cossington Smith painted a portion of the wall, as did Roy de Maistre. We sat there for a time, each with our own thoughts – I was surprised to find myself quite relaxed, quite peaceful …

… Anna's Oscar suddenly cut through, 'When's lunch?!'

So we rose quietly, left the crypt and went outside.

Out into the sunshine.

One year on … a gently placed full stop.

References

I have used, as source material, *A Guide to Painting in Original Settings: VENICE*, by Terisio Pignatti, published in 1995 by Canal and Stamperia Editrice srl, Venezia, and *A Literary Companion: VENICE*, by Ian Littlewood, published by John Murray (Publishers) Ltd, London.

I also wish to acknowledge the following:

The song 'If You Were the Only Girl in the World' by Nat D. Ayer with lyrics by Clifford Grey. It is reproduced with kind permission by J. Albert & Son Pty Ltd. All rights reserved.

The hymn 'The Lord bless and keep you' by John Rutter.

The Beaux Stratagem by George Farquhar, edited with an introduction by W. D. Taylor, published by Oxford University Press.

'The Rime of the Ancient Mariner' by Samuel Taylor Coleridge, presented by Willy Pogámy, published by George G. Harrap & Company Limited, London.

The version of Solomon's *Song of Songs* from the Australian edition of *The Coming of the Cosmic Christ* by Matthew Fox, published by Collins Dove, Melbourne, 1989.

The italicised passages on pages 227 and 231 are by Anna Phillips.

The song 'Wish Me Luck As You Wave Me Good-bye' by Harry David and Phil Park. It is reproduced with kind permission by Warner/Chappell Music, Australia Pty Ltd.

The quotations from *The Tempest* are from the play's Epilogue, from *The Complete Works of William Shakespeare*, with an introduction by St. John Ervine, published by The Literary Press Limited, London.